THE DIURETIC MANUAL

THE DIURETIC MANUAL

Editor

Jules B. Puschett, M.D.

Professor of Medicine
Director, Renal-Electrolyte Division
University of Pittsburgh School of Medicine

Associate Editor

Arthur Greenberg, M.D.

Assistant Professor of Medicine
Member, Renal-Electrolyte Division
University of Pittsburgh School of Medicine

ELSEVIER
New York • Amsterdam • Oxford

NOTICE:
The editors and the publisher of this work have made every effort to ensure that the drug dosage schedules herein are accurate and in accord with the standards accepted at the time of publication. Readers are advised, however, to check the product information sheet included in the package of each drug prior to administration to be certain that changes have not been made in either the recommended doses or contraindications. Such verification is especially important in regard to new or infrequently used drugs.

Elsevier Science Publishing Co., Inc.
52 Vanderbilt Avenue, New York, New York 10017

Sole distributors outside the United States and Canada:

Elsevier Science Publishers B.V.
P.O. Box 211, 1000 AE Amsterdam, The Netherlands

Library of Congress Cataloging in Publication Data

Main entry under title:

The Diuretic manual.

Includes index.
1. Diuretics. I. Puschett, Jules B. II. Greenberg, Arthur.
[DNLM: 1. Diuretics. QV-160 D6169]
RM377.D54 1984 615'.761 84-6143
ISBN 0-444-00879-9

Manufactured in the United States of America

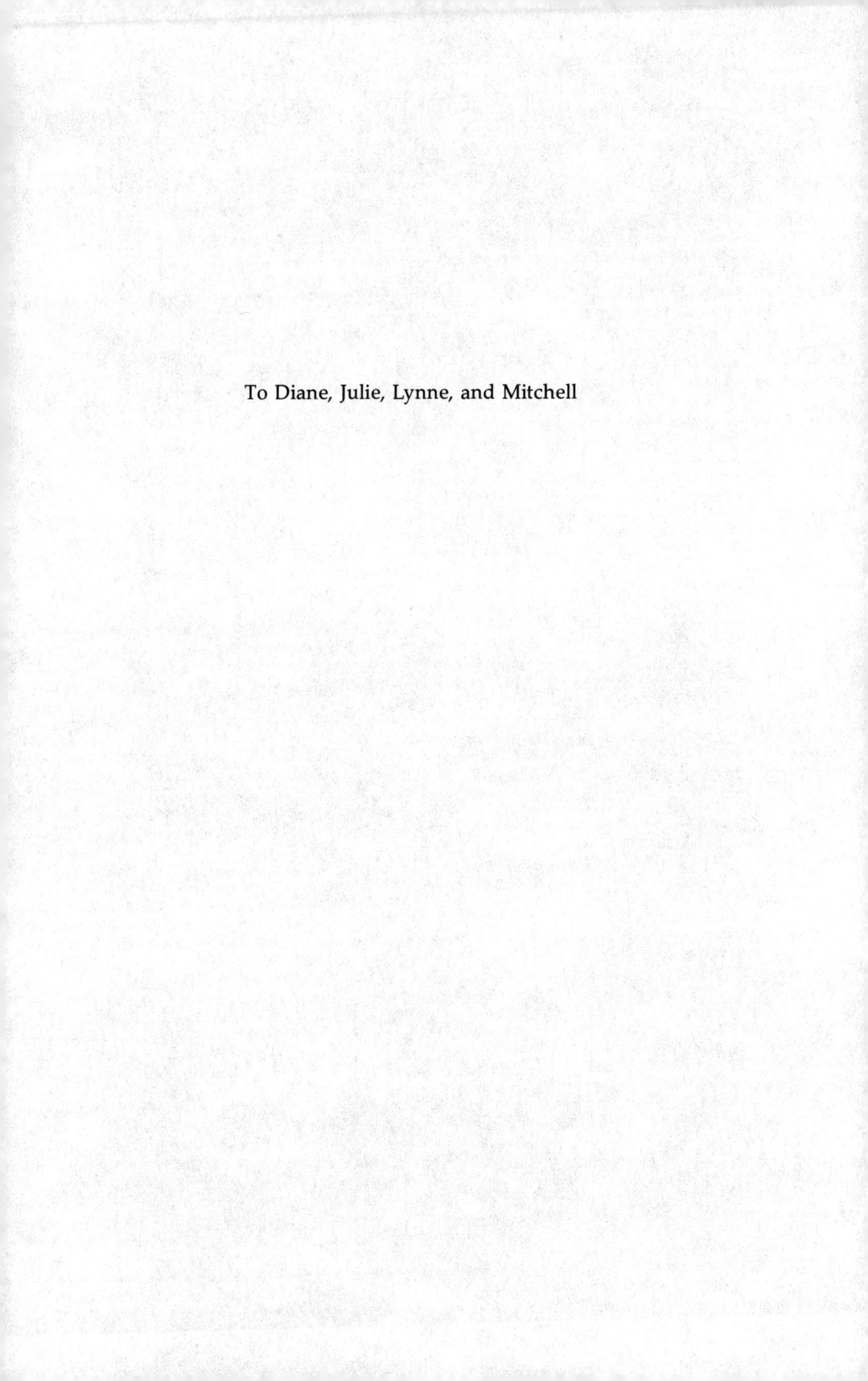

To Diane, Julie, Lynne, and Mitchell

Contents

Foreword

The mid-to-late twentieth century has been marked by dramatic advances in pharmacotherapeutics. The development of drugs such as antibiotics, chemotherapeutic agents, anticoagulants, anesthetics, hypnotics, sedatives, receptor antagonists, analgesics, anti-inflammatory agents, and psychotropic agents, and the purification and synthesis of hormones have changed the practice of medicine and led to the effective treatment and cure of a host of diseases. Progress in the area of diuretic therapy has been equally dramatic and therapeutically successful. A perusal of the history of diuretic therapy serves as a window by which to observe the accretion of knowledge of renal physiology as each new class of diuretics has exerted effects at specific yet different sites in the nephron. For several decades, the mercurial diuretics that acted on the proximal and distal nephron to decrease reabsorption were paramount in the treatment of edematous states. Side effects, including mercury intoxication, agranulocytosis, and sudden death after intravenous injection, limited their use. Carbonic anhydrase inhibitors such as acetazolamide ultimately proved to be weak diuretics but provided great insights into tubular function. These agents, by virtue of their ability to inhibit carbonic anhydrase in the tubular cell, resulted in impaired H^+ secretion and induced urinary sodium, bicarbonate, potassium, and water excretion. Of greatest importance, however, structure-activity studies of carbonic anhydrase inhibitors gave rise most unexpectedly to the class of diuretics known as benzothiadiazides, of which chlorothiazide was the first to be clinically utilized to any significant degree. These agents produce a chloride diuresis and clearly demonstrate the independence of their action on sodium, chloride, and water excretion from the inhibitors of carbonic anhydrase. The property of inducing sodium excretion has also served to establish the benzothiadiazides as the linchpin around which virtually all antihypertensive therapy is based and they have become the prototype of step 1 drugs for the treatment of millions of patients with hypertension. Most recently the "loop" diuretics, including furosemide, ethacrynic acid, and bumetanide, have achieved a prominent place in diuretic therapy. The primary effect of these drugs is to decrease chloride and sodium reabsorption in the ascending limb of the loop of Henle.

The diuretic manual developed by Dr. Puschett and his colleagues provides an indepth discussion of the many uses of modern diuretics including therapy of edematous states found in a variety of clinical disorders, management of hypertension, and adjunctive therapy of patients with absorptive hypercalciurias and renal stones. Extensive discussion is provided regarding the modern concepts of renal physiology in order for the reader to understand the action of specific types of diuretics. The section on diuretic site and mechanism of action serves to highlight the sophisticated technologies presently utilized in the study of renal physiology and mechanism of diuretic action which are providing fundamental insights into the molecular biology of renal tubular cells.

Based on the data presented in this manual, it seems clear that the next decade will most likely witness the development of additional diuretic agents specifically tailored to intervene in the basic biochemical reactions that are responsible for the characteristic and complex transport systems for water and solute in the various parts of the human nephron. The rapid evolution of diuretic therapy over the past quarter century and the excitement of the present state-of-the-art justifiably lead to considerable anticipation for the advances of the future.

Gerald S. Levey, M.D.

Pittsburgh, Pennsylvania

Preface

Diuretics are among the most heavily utilized therapeutic agents in clinical medicine. Despite this fact, there is no single source to which the clinician can refer which provides, in one volume, suggestions for their employment in various disease entities, as well as the physiologic and pharmacologic bases for their administration. This book represents an attempt by my colleagues and me to provide this sort of information. In Part I, chapters 1–13, we have detailed specific suggestions for therapy in eleven types of disorders and/or special patient populations. In each chapter, these recommendations follow concise introductory material with regard to the establishment of a diagnosis and a review of what is currently known about pathogenesis. Furthermore, potential complications and important drug interactions of the diuretics are presented. Some repetition of salient points will be noted, as we recognize that our readers may not have time to peruse every chapter. It is hoped that Part I will be of use to practicing physicians of all kinds, but especially to general practitioners, general internists, nephrologists, and cardiologists. House officers may also find the practical aspects of these chapters helpful in their day-to-day management of patients.

Chapter 14 outlines the renal physiologic principles upon which sound therapeutic decisions are based. Accordingly, this portion of the book should prove to be of interest to medical students as well as to those physicians who have a more compelling interest in understanding how and why diuretics work. Part II appendixes consisting of several special topics. The commercially available diuretics are listed, classified as to their relative potencies, their major and minor sites of action within the nephron and the indications for their use.

It is appropriate, at this juncture, to thank my colleagues who have so unselfishly given of their time, which I recognize included many evenings and weekends of work. I also thank their wives, husbands, and children, who had less time with them because of their contributions to this book. We are all grateful to the secretarial staff of the Renal-Electrolyte Division of the University of Pittsburgh School of Medicine who have toiled so diligently to produce the manuscript. My special thanks to my Associate Editor, Dr. Arthur Greenberg, who has not only contributed importantly to these pages, but has collated and reviewed all of the material contained herein.

Jules B. Puschett, M.D.

Pittsburgh, Pennsylvania

Contributors

Ellis Avner, M.D.
Assistant Professor of Pediatrics, University of Pittsburgh School of Medicine; Staff Nephrologist, Children's Hospital of Pittsburgh

Barbara Carpenter, M.D.
Assistant Professor of Medicine, Member, Renal-Electrolyte Division, University of Pittsburgh School of Medicine

Jesus Dominguez, M.D.
Assistant Professor of Medicine, Member, Renal-Electrolyte Division, University of Pittsburgh School of Medicine

Demetrius Ellis, M.D.
Assistant Professor of Pediatrics, University of Pittsburgh School of Medicine; Director, Division of Nephrology, Children's Hospital of Pittsburgh

Arthur Greenberg, M.D.
Assistant Professor of Medicine, Member, Renal-Electrolyte Division, University of Pittsburgh School of Medicine

Patricia D. Kroboth, Ph.D.
Assistant Professor of Pharmacy Practice and Medicine, University of Pittsburgh Schools of Pharmacy and Medicine

Gerald S. Levey, M.D.
Professor and Chairman, Department of Medicine, University of Pittsburgh School of Medicine

Beth Piraino, M.D.
Assistant Professor of Medicine, Member, Renal-Electrolyte Division, University of Pittsburgh School of Medicine

Thomas O. Pitts, M.D.
Assistant Professor of Medicine, Member, Renal-Electrolyte Division, University of Pittsburgh School of Medicine

Jules B. Puschett, M.D.
Professor of Medicine, Director, Renal-Electrolyte Division, University of Pittsburgh School of Medicine

Raymond Rault, M.D.
Assistant Professor of Medicine, Member, Renal-Electrolyte Division, University of Pittsburgh School of Medicine

Marcia Silver, M.D.
Assistant Professor of Medicine, Member, Renal-Electrolyte Division, University of Pittsburgh School of Medicine

Michael Sorkin, M.D.
Assistant Professor of Medicine, Member, Renal-Electrolyte Division, University of Pittsburgh School of Medicine

PART

I

DIURETIC THERAPY PHYSIOLOGIC BASIS AND CLINICAL ASPECTS

chapter

1

Edema Formation and the Physiologic Basis for Diuretic Usage

An Introduction

Jules B. Puschett, M.D.

With the exception of those edema states which represent local phenomena (for example, related to venous stasis), the final common pathway by which edema occurs is the perception by the kidney of some signal or series of stimuli, that cause(s) the retention of salt and water. This may be appropriate and salutary in the patient with hemorrhagic shock. On the other hand, this response of the kidney to enhance sodium reabsorption may be inimical to the patient's best interests, as in the patient with congestive heart failure, who often already has an expanded extracellular fluid volume. Therefore, what the congestive heart failure and hemorrhagic shock patient have in common with the patients suffering from ascites and/or edema due to hepatic disease or the nephrotic syndrome, is an apparent hypoperfusion of the renal vascular bed. While not entirely understood, the pathogenesis of these disorders probably includes alterations in the physical forces which regulate transport across the glomerular capillaries ("glomerular factors"), and those involved in the post-glomerular circulation, which regulate tubular reabsorption ("tubular factors"). In addition, one or more humoral mechanisms may be involved. Diuretics are substances which act to impair sodium transport within the tubular system, leading to an increased excretion of sodium ions with an attendant anion, which carry with them filtered water. In certain special circumstances, diuretics may act, in part, not by altering tubular ionic reabsorption, but by raising filtered sodium load through the mechanism of increasing renal blood flow and glomerular filtration rate (GFR). An example of this type of diuretic agent is the xanthine class of drugs e.g., theophylline. Table 1.1 presents a list of drugs which can act as diuretic agents. It will be noted that some of them, such as digitalis glycosides, can have both glomerular and tubular effects.

TABLE 1-1. Mechanisms of Action of Drugs Capable of Diuretic Effects

Drug	Presumed Mechanism of Effect
1. Drugs Which Enhance the Filtered Load of Sodium	
a. Xanthine derivatives (theophylline, etc.)	a. ↑ Renal blood flow due to afferent arteriolar vasodilatation
b. Dopamine	b. ↓ Renal vascular resistance, ↑ renal blood flow
c. Dobutamine	c. ↑ Cardiac contractility and ↑ cardiac output
d. Digitalis glycosides	d. Augment renal perfusion by improving cardiac output
2. Drugs Which Impair Tubular Reabsorption[a]	
a. Acetazolamide	a. Carbonic anhydrase inhibition
b. Thiazides	b. Unknown; additional proximal effect, if any, thought to be due to carbonic anhydrase inhibition
c. Metolazone	c. Unknown; proximal effect (seen only with loop blockade) not due to carbonic anhydrase inhibition
d. Furosemide	d. Unknown
e. Ethacrynic acid	e. Unknown
f. Bumetanide	f. Unknown
g. Mercurials	g. Intrarenal release of mercuric ions by rupture of C-Hg bonds with capture of thiol groups
h. Spironolactone	h. Competitive inhibition of tubular effects of aldosterone
i. Triamterene	i. Unknown (direct inhibitory effect on potassium secretion)
j. Amiloride	j. Unknown
k. Digitalis glycosides	k. Inhibition of Na^+-K^+ ATPase

[a]See also Part II (Appendix 2).

Physiologic Principles

An understanding of the formation of edema and the potential utility of diuretics in the management of this abnormality is based upon certain physiologic principles regarding glomerular and tubular function. In order for edema formation to occur, the patient must excrete less sodium than he is taking in. In other words, positive sodium and water balance must occur. The excretion of sodium can decline leading to positive sodium balance, either because the filtered load of sodium is reduced or because tubular reabsorption is increased, or both. Theoretically, therapy should be aimed at raising filtered load or reducing tubular reabsorption, or both. As a practical matter, it is usually difficult or impossible to increase the filtered load of sodium which has been abnormally lowered by a disease process. Thus, for the most part, treatment is directed toward inhibiting the tubular transport of sodium. In some cases, therapy can also be aimed at a reversal of the underlying pathophysiologic process. Examples of the latter include: an improvement in cardiac output in the patient with congestive heart failure, thus re-establishing normal or near-normal renal perfusion and glomerular filtration rate; or, therapy of glomerular disease in patients with nephrotic syndrome, leading to the correction of abnormal physical forces across the glomerular capillaries.

Glomerular Factors

Filtered load essentially depends upon GFR alone as this ion is not protein bound and since plasma sodium concentration varies very little except in unusual circumstances. The ability of the kidney to filter solute is a function of the hydrostatic pressure in the glomerular capillaries which, in turn, is a function of the blood pressure (Figure 1-1). The glomerular hydrostatic pressure favors filtration; this force is opposed by the plasma oncotic pressure as well as by the intratubular pressure. This relationship can be quantified and has been measured in the experimental animal.

If we define SNGFR as the filtration rate of a single filtering unit of the kidney or nephron, and K_f as the ultrafiltration coefficient, and $\bar{P}_{uf}$ as the net force for ultrafiltration, then

$$SNGFR = K_f \times \bar{P}_{uf}.$$

Since $\bar{P}_{uf}$, is in turn the difference ($\overline{\Delta P}$) between the mean hydrostatic pressure drop across the glomerular capillary and the difference ($\Delta \bar{\pi}$) between glomerular capillary and Bowman's space colloid oncotic pressure (1), it is clear that

$$SNGFR = K_f\ (\overline{\Delta P} - \Delta \bar{\pi}).$$

Since K_f is the product of the hydraulic permeability of the capillary wall (K) and the total surface available for filtration (S)

$$SNGFR = K \times S \times \bar{P}_{uf}.$$

It has been determined that in addition to the major role that K_f, $\overline{\Delta P}$ and $\overline{\Delta \pi}$ play in the determination of SNGFR, glomerular plasma flow rate (Q_A) also exerts a considerable influence. SNGFR is directly related to Q_A by an expression which includes the single nephron filtration fraction (SNFF) as follows:

$$SNFF = SNGFR/Q_A.$$

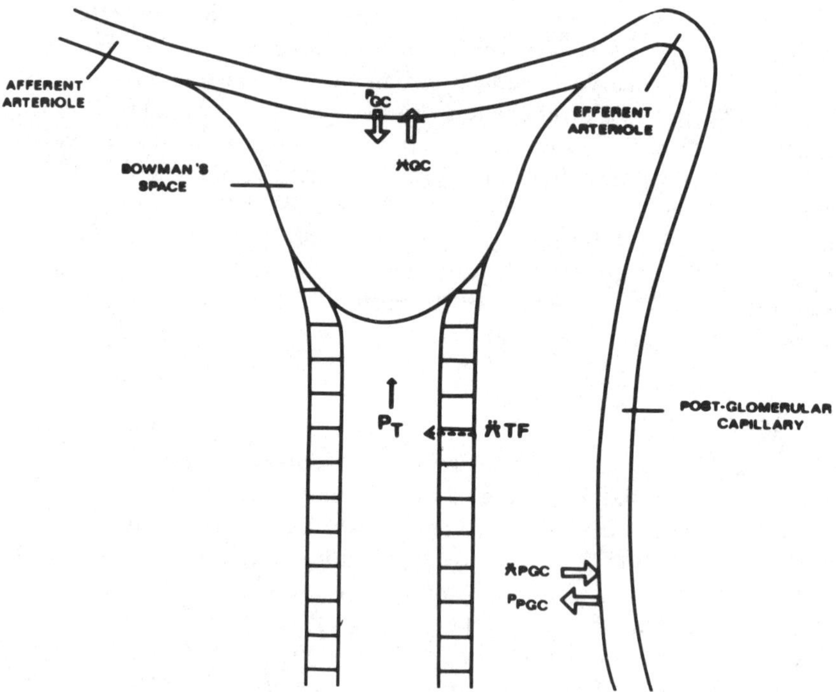

Figure 1-1. The physical forces which regulate glomerular filtration include P_{GC}, the glomerular capillary hydrostatic pressure, the main force for ultrafiltration, and the glomerular capillary oncotic pressure ($\bar{\pi}$ GC), which is the major force opposing filtration. Pressure in Bowman's space and in the tubular system (P_T) also opposes filtration but, except in the circumstance of tubular obstruction, is usually so small as to be negligible. Proximal tubular reabsorption depends in a major way on the interplay of physical forces across the post-glomerular circulation. Here, the post-glomerular capillary oncotic pressure ($\bar{\pi}$PGC) is an important factor favoring reabsorption, and is opposed by hydrostatic pressure in the post-glomerular capillary (P_{PGC}), which is usually small. Any oncotic force due to protein in the tubular lumen ($\bar{\pi}$TF) would also retard reabsorption, but this force probably only becomes of any significance in advanced disease states. Active transport of sodium forms the major force moving proximal tubular fluid and electrolytes from tubular lumen to capillary blood.

The SNFF represents that portion of the blood coursing through the glomerulus (Q_A) that becomes glomerular ultrafiltrate (SNGFR). Rearrangement of the equation yields:

$$SNGFR = SNFF \times Q_A,$$

demonstrating the direct relationship between glomerular plasma flow (Q_A) and single nephron filtration rate.

Given these physical relationships, it is possible to extrapolate from data obtained in the experimental animal, in which direct measurements of the parameters outlined above have been made, to human disease states. Thus, SNGFR might fall, reducing filtered load, because K_f is reduced (as is probably the case in glomerulonephritis) (2,3), or because hydraulic pressure and/or Q_A is (are) reduced (as in shock states). It should be obvious, therefore, that in the treatment of edematous patients, attention should be given to the correction of the underlying abnormality, if this is at all possible.

Tubular Factors

Similar considerations to those outlined above regarding the physical forces that determine glomerular ultrafiltration also pertain to the reabsorption of fluid and electrolytes from the tubular system. The best studied of these areas is the proximal convoluted tubule (Figure 1-2). In health, the reabsorption of fluid and sodium proximally appears to be a function of tubular flow rate as well as the hydraulic and oncotic pressure relationships that exist across the post-glomerular peritubular capillary. If flow rate in the tubule increases, fluid and sodium reabsorption increase (4) and the reverse is also probably true. Therefore, the tubular system adjusts for alterations in glomerular filtration rate by varying absolute salt and water reabsorption, with the result that *fractional* reabsorption remains constant. This maintenance of the fractional reabsorptive rate has been termed "glomerulotubular balance." Abnormalities in renal function or the imposition of marked variations in extracellular fluid volume (either volume expansion or marked volume contraction) tend to disrupt glomerulotubular balance, leading to alterations in the fractional excretion of salt and water.

The effect of physical factors on transtubular reabsorption of salt and water is largely a function of peritubular capillary hydrostatic pressure and protein concentration. For example, if there is a reduction in renal blood flow (RBF) without a fall in GFR or if RBF falls more than GFR, then filtration fraction will rise and so will the concentration of protein in the peritubular capillary. The latter change will tend to enhance proximal tubular reabsorption (Figure 1-1). Such a sequence of events has been proposed to explain the pathophysiology of edema formation in a number of clinical situations in which hypoperfusion is thought to occur, such as congestive heart failure and persistent hypotension.

Finally, with regard to tubular function, evidence has accrued which suggests that, at least under some circumstances, a natriuretic hormonal

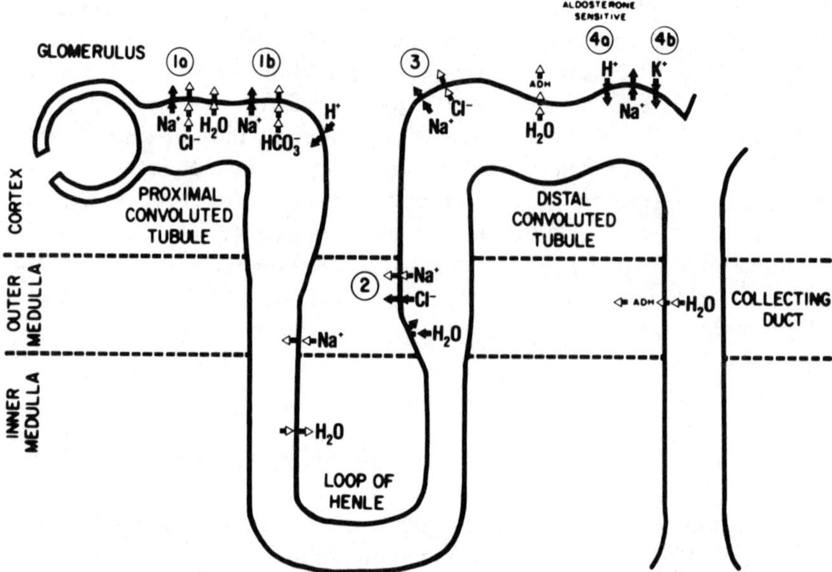

Figure 1-2. Nephron sites of electrolyte and fluid reabsorption. The proximal nephron loci have been designated 1a and 1b to differentiate between sodium chloride (1a) and sodium bicarbonate (1b) reabsorption. Similarly, site 4a represents aldosterone-regulated Na-H-K exchange while site 4b depicts the portion of this transfer process not under the control of the mineralocorticoids. See text for additional explanation. *Reproduced from Cardiovascular Medicine 2: 119–134, 1977, by permission of the editors.*

factor may be elaborated. This was first suggested when it became clear that the natriuresis of volume expansion could not be accounted for entirely on the basis of alterations in the filtered load of sodium and/or on changes in mineralocorticoid control of distal tubular sodium exchange (5). It has been postulated that the putative natriuretic or "third" factor is of importance in uremia (6), and possibly also in essential hypertension (7). Whether deficiency of such a hormone accounts, at least in part, for the antidiuresis and antinatriuresis seen in such clinical situations as advanced hepatic disease associated with ascites and edema, remains entirely speculative at this point.

Profile of Tubular Function by Nephron Site

As discussed earlier in this chapter, both glomerular and tubular factors may be involved in edema formation. However, practically speaking, diuretics are seldom given to enhance filtered sodium load, but rather are utilized largely to inhibit tubular sodium reabsorption. To understand diuretic mechanisms and sites of action, it is important to review normal tubular function. Presented in Figure 1-2 are the major loci at which sodium and water transport are accomplished in the nephron (8). In the proximal tubule, which consists of both convoluted and straight portions, it has been estimated that 60–70% of salt and water are reabsorbed. Sodium transport is active in this segment. Furthermore, water is reabsorbed isotonically at this nephron site. In addition, the majority of the phosphate and 80–90% of bicarbonate are reabsorbed proximally. According to current concepts, potassium is virtually completely reabsorbed early in the nephron and that which appears in the final urine is added to the tubular contents in the late distal nephron.

The clinical implications of these physiologic principles are as follows: First, although the major portion of sodium is reabsorbed in the proximal nephron segment, interference by a diuretic with sodium reabsorption in this portion of the nephron does not assure that the drug will be a potent natriuretic agent. This is because sodium ions which are rejected proximally by virtue of the drug's action on tubular transport can be reabsorbed in the distal nephron. Acetazolamide (Diamox) causes a considerable reduction of proximal sodium reabsorption by virtue of its ability to impair sodium bicarbonate transport, yet is only a mildly to moderately potent diuretic (see Part II, Appendix 1). As most of the phosphate and bicarbonate ions which are filtered are reabsorbed proximally, their excretion pattern is of importance to renal physiologists and pharmacologists as a "marker" of proximal function. Therefore, if a diuretic drug causes a major phosphaturia and bicarbonate diuresis, it is likely that wherever else it acts within the nephron, it has a significant proximal effect.

As the tubular fluid leaves the proximal nephron segment, it enters the loop of Henle. While the transport properties of the descending limb and hairpin turn of the loop of Henle are crucial in understanding the countercurrent system, the solute and water transport that occur in this nephron segment are not of great magnitude. Therefore, we can proceed to consider the function of the ascending limb of the loop of Henle, especially that of the thick outer medullary portion (site 2, Figure 1-2). At this nephron site, chloride appears to be the actively transported moiety with sodium following passively. Approximately 20–30% of filtered sodium is reabsorbed at this locus. Furthermore, the loop of Henle seems to have a rather capacious transport mechanism, as the presentation to it of large increments of NaCl results in a rather consistent increase in absolute reabsorption (9). It is at this site that the potent diuretics furosemide (Lasix), ethacrynic acid (Edecrin), and bumetanide (Bumex) exert their major effects. If an agent blocks salt transport at this site in the nephron, its chances of causing a major natriuresis are good for two reasons: 1) The drug is inhibiting sodium reabsorption in an area of the nephron that is closer to the end of the tubular stream. Ions rejected at the level of the loop of Henle have only to escape reabsorption in the distal tubule and collecting duct to appear in the final urine (see Figure 1-2). Because the more distal transport sites have limited capacities, ions rejected by the loop of Henle have an excellent opportunity to be excreted by the kidney. 2) In addition, loop diuretics are effective in a segment of the nephron that reabsorbs significant amounts of sodium chloride.

Whereas ions and water are transported isotonically in the proximal tubule, in the ascending limb of the loop of Henle their reabsorptive characteristics diverge. The tubular epithelium of the thick ascending limb behaves as if it is essentially "water tight." Therefore, in this nephron segment, solute (mainly NaCl) leaves the tubular lumen, whereas tubular water remains behind (Figure 1-2). Accordingly, the tubular contents are diluted, and solute-free water ("free water") is generated. Interference with sodium chloride reabsorption at this transport site (by the loop diuretics) can therefore impair free water formation and could result in hyponatremia (see Chapter 10).

In the early reaches of the distal convoluted tubule is a transport site at which another 5–10% of the filtered sodium is reabsorbed by an active transport process (site 3, Figure 1-2). It is at this site that the thiazides, metolazone (Zaroxolyn) and chlorthalidone (Hygroton), are thought to have their effects. In the late portion of the distal convolution and probably also located in the collecting duct, is a specialized transport mechanism at which sodium is exchanged for hydrogen and potassium, rather than being transported with an accompanying anion. Only a portion of the function of this site is under the control of aldosterone. That is, sodium can still be exchanged despite the absence of adrenal function, although the transport capacity is reduced. These two mechanisms are labeled sites 4a and 4b, respectively, in Figure 1-2. Spironolactone (Aldactone) competitively inhibits aldosterone and is therefore effective at site 4a, while triamterene (Dyrenium) and amiloride (Midamor) have a direct effect to impair hydrogen and potassium excretion (site 4b). Sodium transport at site 4 rarely exceeds 2–3% of filtered load. Accordingly, those diuretics that are effective in blocking sodium reabsorption at site 4 are not given primarily because of their diuretic and natriuretic potency, but because they tend to limit or decrease potassium excretion. When one employs these so-called potassium-sparing agents in patients, the following important clinical considerations should be recognized. First, when potassium secretion is inhibited by these drugs, so is hydrogen ion secretion. Accordingly, it is important to remember that the development of hyperkalemic metabolic acidosis is a possibility, especially in patients who have renal insufficiency, and who may already be having problems excreting potassium and hydrogen ion. Any diuretic which acts anywhere in the nephron proximal to site 4, thereby presenting more sodium to that transport site, will increase the secretion of potassium into the tubular fluid (10). The hallmark of a potent natriuretic agent is its tendency to produce a kaliuresis. In general, the more potent a natriuretic agent, the greater will be the kaliuresis it causes, and the greater the tendency to produce hypokalemia (see Figure 1-3).

As was the case for the loop of Henle, electrolyte and water transport are regulated separately in the distal convoluted tubule and collecting duct. In these portions of the nephron, water reabsorption occurs if antidiuretic hormone (ADH) is present. The force for this water reabsortion is the osmotic gradient generated by the pumping of salt (and urea) into the medullary interstitium, especially by the loop of Henle (site 2, Figure 1-2). The countercurrent system in the renal medulla functions to establish and maintain this hypertonic gradient. If ADH has been suppressed, then

Figure 1-3. Changes in the percentage excretion rate of potassium ($\Delta C_K/C_{In} \times 100$) as a function of the increment in percentage sodium excretion ($\Delta C_{Na}/C_{In} \times 100$) produced by five diuretic agents. The studies were performed in normal volunteers. Although the degree of kaliuresis obtained for a given degree of natriuresis differs for each drug, nevertheless, in general, the greater the natriuretic potency of the agent, the greater the tendency to induce a kaliuresis. *Key:* ○ Acetazolamide, ● Chlorothiazide, ■ Furosemide, □ ECA, and ▲ Metolazone. *Reprinted from Clin. Pharm. Ther. 15: 397–405, 1974, with permission of the editors.*

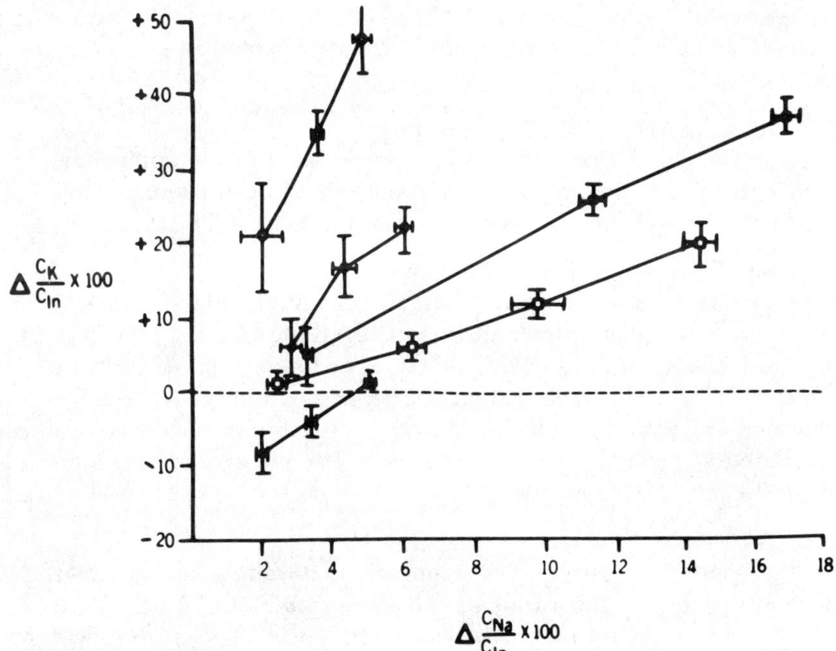

water reabsorption from the distal tubule and collecting duct is impaired, and a dilute urine is elaborated. Furthermore, if a diuretic inhibits the transport of sodium chloride into the renal medulla, it interferes with the concentrating process since the ability of the kidney to form a hypertonic medulla is compromised.

Resistant Edema

The development of a truly resistant edema state is a rather uncommon clinical circumstance. In general, this situation results from one or more of the following:

1. *Reduced Glomerular Filtration Rate*

If the GFR has been markedly reduced, either by a dramatic reduction in renal blood flow or for other reasons, there will be a decreased delivery of filtrate to the tubular system. Under these circumstances, even if the diuretic agent is able to inhibit transport, the magnitude of the sodium transport impairment may be so small as to limit any natriuresis or diuresis.

2. *Marked Increase in Proximal Reabsorption*

In clinical states characterized by renal hypoperfusion (e.g., congestive heart failure, hemorrhagic shock, etc.), the kidney responds in a very primitive way to augment proximal reabsorption. In advanced disease, therefore, inhibition of sodium reabsorption by diuretics which act in the loop of Henle or beyond (see Figure 1-2) will be ineffectual in inducing a diuresis.

3. *Altered Renal Tubular Architecture*

In order for a diuretic to work, an intact tubular epithelium and transport mechanism are required. If these have been badly damaged by anatomic changes, then it is unlikely that the drug will be effective.

4. *Reduced Bioavailability of the Drug*

It appears that diuretic agents must obtain entrance to the tubular lumen in order to impair transepithelial transport. If the blood supply is greatly reduced, insufficient drug may gain contact with the luminal surface of the renal tubular cell for its action to become manifest. Alternatively, if diuretics are given to patients who have edema of the intestinal wall (in addition to edema elsewhere), the patient may not absorb sufficient drug from the gut to have an effect.

5. *Acid–Base Disturbances*

a) Metabolic acidosis—the development of metabolic acidosis interferes with the ability of the carbonic anhydrase inhibitors to act as diuretic agents. This is because this class of diuretics acts by interfering with the "reabsorption" of bicarbonate, resulting in the excretion of sodium ions which accompany bicarbonate into the urine. If the filtered load of bicarbonate is low, as is the case in metabolic acidosis, in which the serum level of bicarbonate is reduced, then the blockade of bicarbonate reabsorption will have a diminished efficacy in producing a natriuresis.

b) Metabolic alkalosis—low serum chloride and high bicarbonate (as occurs in metabolic alkalosis) appear to impair the ability of the mercurial diuretics to induce a natriuresis. While the exact mechanism of this effect is unknown, this "resistance" to mercurial diuretics can be overcome by pretreating the patient with ammonium chloride.

Therapy of resistant edema should be approached physiologically. If the patient's GFR is markedly reduced (less than about 10 ml/min), chances are that diuretics will no longer be effective. If, on the other hand, one suspects that resistance is related to enhanced proximal reabsorption, sodium transport blockade at multiple sites in the nephron may be warranted and effective. For example, impairment of sodium reabsorption in the loop of Henle should be attempted, and then a proximally active drug should be given, so that proximally rejected ions can be delivered past the transport site in the ascending limb of the loop of Henle. In some cases, a third agent could be given: for example, blockade of the sodium-hydrogen-potassium (Na-H-K) site in the late distal nephron and collecting duct (see Figure 1-2) could be attempted. A regimen which has proved useful in the author's experience is the oral administration of metolazone (5–10 mg) followed in about 1 hr by the intravenous injection of furosemide (up to 240 mg) or bumetanide (up to 3–5 mg). Other combinations of agents may also be worthwhile (see Appendix 2 for sites of action).

General Guidelines for Diuretic Therapy

Although diuretic therapy must be tailored to the individual patient, the following general guidelines have proved useful to the author and his colleagues in the therapy of edema states.

1. As with all other drugs, diuretics should be given orally rather than intravenously, except when IV drug is indicated, as follows: a) in emergency situations (e.g., acute pulmonary edema), or b) when gastrointestinal absorption is uncertain or impaired (gut wall edema, rapid GI transit time, naso-gastric suction, etc.)
2. Give the smallest effective dose, and repeat that dose when the urine flow rate declines, if the diuretic goal has not been achieved. It should be emphasized that one must first find the effective dose by incrementing the amount of drug given on a single occasion. Once that dose has been established, one can then repeat it as needed to achieve the therapeutic response that is desired. For example, if a patient has responded poorly to 40 mg of furosemide in the morning,

80 mg should be administered next time, rather than repeating the 40 mg dose later in the day.

3. When it is determined that the patient is not responding to large doses of orally administered diuretics and it is decided to switch to intravenous drug, the dose must be dramatically reduced. Thus, patients with gut wall edema who have not responded to 240 mg of furosemide p.o., for example, will often have a dramatic natriuresis from 40 mg (or even 20 mg) given IV. Adherence to this principle will result in the avoidance of massive natriuresis with its attendant complications. One can always give more IV drug, but once it is in the circulation, it cannot be retrieved.
4. Kaliuretic tendency is a function of natriuretic potency (see above). Therefore, hypokalemia should be expected and treated when a major natriuresis is induced.
5. The commonest acid-base disturbance caused by diuretics is hypokalemic metabolic alkalosis (see also Chapter 10). This disorder results from the fact that sodium is excreted largely with chloride, rather than bicarbonate, and because potassium depletion results in the exchange of sodium for hydrogen ion at the distal nephron exchange site (Figure 1-2). Correction of this disturbance involves the provision of potassium as the *chloride,* not as potassium bicarbonate (or bicarbonate equivalent, such as the gluconate). Therapy with the bicarbonate salt will perpetuate the acid-base disorder and will make it difficult to replete total body potassium.
6. Diuretic resistance is better treated by blocking sodium transport at more than one site in the nephron (that is, by combined drug therapy) than by getting involved with heroic doses of a single drug. The latter practice generally is not only not effective, but also places the patient in jeopardy for the development of those side effects of the diuretics which are not usually seen when lower doses are given (see Chapter 10). For example, we rarely exceed 240 mg of furosemide as a single dose.
7. It is axiomatic that diuretics should not be given to patients who are volume contracted. If the patient is hypovolemic or if the status of the extracellular fluid volume is unknown, then a trial of volume expansion should be given first. Once repletion of the ECF volume has been assured, diuretics can be tried cautiously, if oliguria persists.

References

1. Brenner, B.M. Glomerular filtration. In: The Kidney, 2nd edition, 1981 (editors: B.M. Brenner and F.C. Rector, Jr.), Philadelphia, W.B. Saunders Co., pp. 289–327.

2. Blantz, R.C., and Wilson, C.B. Acute effects of antiglomerular basement membrane antibody on the process of glomerular filtration in the rat. J. Clin. Invest. 58:899–911, 1976.

3. Maddox, D.A., Bennett, C.H., Dunn, W.M., Glassock, R.J., Knutson, D., Daugherty, T.M., and Brenner, B.M. Determinants of glomerular filtration in experimental glomerulonephritis in the rat. J. Clin. Invest. 55:305–318, 1975.

4. Häberle, D., and von Baeyer, H. Characteristics of glomerulotubular balance. Am. J. Physiol. 244:F355–366, 1983.

5. de Wardener, H.E., Mills, I.H., Clapham, W.F., and Hayter, C.J. Studies on the efferent mechanism of the sodium diuresis which follows the administration of intravenous saline in the dog. Clin. Sci. 21:249–258, 1961.

6. Bourgoignie, J.J., Hwang, K.H., Espinel, C., Klahr, S., and Bricker, N.S. A natriuretic factor in the serum of patients with chronic uremia. J. Clin. Invest. 51:1514–1527, 1972.

7. de Wardener, H.E., and MacGregor, G.A. Dahl's hypothesis that a saliuretic substance may be responsible for a sustained rise in arterial pressure: its possible role in essential hypertension. Kidney Int. 18:1–9, 1980.

8. Puschett, J.B. Physiologic basis for the use of new and older diuretics in congestive heart failure. Cardiovascular Medicine 2:119–134, 1977.

9. Buckalew, V.M., Jr., Walker, B.R., Puschett, J.B., and Goldberg, M. Effects of increased sodium delivery on distal tubular sodium reabsorption with and without volume expansion in man. J. Clin. Invest. 49:2336–2344, 1970.

10. Puschett, J.B., and Rastegar, A. Comparative study of the effects of metolazone and other diuretics on potassium excretion. Clin. Pharm. Ther. 15:397–405, 1974.

chapter

2

Therapy of the Edema Due to the Nephrotic Syndrome

Jules B. Puschett, M.D.

Diagnosis

The nephrotic syndrome represents a complex of symptoms and signs which, in its full-blown form, includes the following diagnostic criteria:

1. Excretion of more than 3–3.5 gm of protein in the urine per 24 hr.
2. A consequent reduction in serum protein (especially albumin) concentration.
3. Hyperlipidemia.
4. Edema.

Pathogenesis

It is clear that the initial event in the pathogenesis of the nephrotic syndrome is the development of an abnormal permeability in the glomerular basement membrane to the passage of circulating plasma proteins, which then leak into the urine. When the ability of the liver to manufacture new plasma protein to replace that which is lost and catabolized is exceeded, the patient goes into negative balance and the serum levels of the protein, especially albumin, fall. Edema develops on at least two bases: 1) a reduction in the circulating level of plasma protein reduces plasma oncotic pressure, allowing fluid to become sequestered in the interstitium (Figure 1) and 2) the development of edema has as its final common pathway the reception of some signal or series of stimuli which causes the kidney to increase its reabsorption of salt and water. This occurs despite the fact that the result of this response on the part of the kidney will be the formation of edema or an increase in the edema already present. In patients with the nephrotic syndrome who have reduced levels

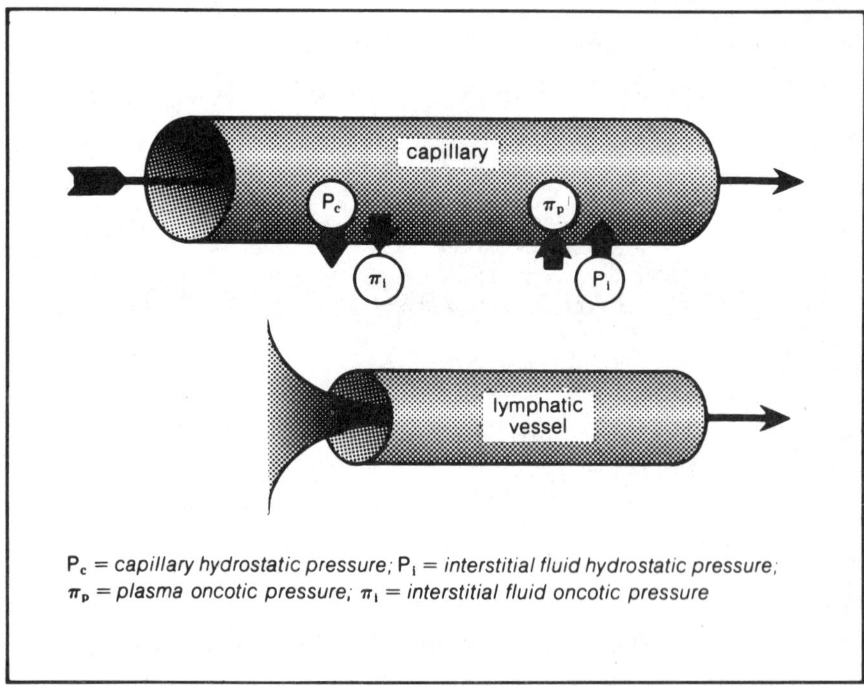

Figure 2-1. Forces governing the distribution of fluid between intravascular and interstitial spaces. *Reproduced with permission, from Cardiovascular Medicine 3:475–488, 1978.*

of GFR, animal models suggest that the decline in SNGFR is due to reductions in renal plasma flow and in K_f (glomerular hydraulic permeability; see Chapter 1) (1, 2). While the development of secondary hyperaldosteronism has been implicated in the formation of the edema seen in this disease state, an important contribution by the renin–angiotensin–aldosterone axis has been difficult to demonstrate in the experimental animal (2). Current thought about the site of the abnormally enhanced reabsorption of salt and water by the kidney based upon animal experimentation, suggests that it occurs either in the collecting ducts and terminal portions of the nephron or that there is an augmentation of reabsorption somewhere along the course of the deep (juxtamedullary) nephrons of the kidney (2, 3), or both.

Differential Diagnosis

Efforts at differential diagnosis are directed toward first verifying the diagnosis of nephrotic syndrome and then determining its etiology, if possible. With regard to the former, it should be apparent from the discussion of pathophysiology (see above) that the complete syndrome may not be present simply because not enough time has elapsed for hypoalbuminemia and edema to have developed. Therefore, one frequently encounters the term "nephrotic range proteinuria" utilized to describe patients who are early in the course of their disease process. It should be emphasized, however, that once the pattern of excretion of large amounts of plasma protein has been established, the patient will usually develop the other diagnostic criteria, unless the disease process remits.

1. *Diagnostic procedures*

a) Urinalysis. Aside from a positive qualitative test for protein, fat droplets may be seen and "Maltese crosses" can often be demonstrated under polarized light. A positive test for sugar would suggest diabetic nephropathy as the etiology of the syndrome, although renal glycosuria may be present in some other forms of renal disease. Red cells and red cell casts suggest underlying glomerulopathy.

b) Twenty-four hr urine collection is used to determine creatinine clearance and total protein excretion. Creatinine is usually reported as mg%. To calculate the clearance,

1. convert urinary creatinine concentration given in mg% to mg/ml by multiplying by 100.
2. multiply this concentration by 24-hr urine volume in ml to get mg of creatinine excreted in 24 hr.
3. divide by 1440 (min in 24 hr) to get mg of creatinine excreted/min.
4. divide the serum creatinine value by 100 to convert from mg% to mg/ml and divide it into the number obtained in (3) to get creatinine clearance in ml/min. Normal values for endogenous creatinine clearance are:*

$$\text{males: } 130 \pm 18 \text{ ml/min/1.73 m}^2$$

$$\text{females: } 120 \pm 14 \text{ ml/min/1.73 m}^2$$

To ascertain the adequacy of the urine collection, divide total creatinine excreted (mg% multiplied by 100, multiplied by total volume of the urine specimen in ml) by the patient's weight in kg. Normal values are:

males: 20–30 mg/kg,

females: 15–25 mg/kg.

---

*There is some disagreement as to whether the values given (which represent inulin clearance) differ for creatinine; current consensus is that the values using the two substances either agree or are only about 7% higher for creatinine clearance (4).

c) Obtain serum albumin and globulin levels.

d) Obtain measurements of plasma lipids.

Determination of the total amount of protein excreted per 24 hr is often used for differential diagnostic purposes as well as to establish the diagnosis of nephrotic syndrome. While patients with glomerular disease may have only small amounts of protein in the urine, patients with interstitial nephropathy usually do not excrete more than 2 grams of protein per 24 hr and rarely more than 3 grams/24 hr. One exception to this rule has recently been described. It consists of patients treated with non-steroidal anti-inflammatory drugs who develop renal insufficiency and nephrotic range proteinuria. On biopsy, they have an acute interstitial nephritis and glomerular basement membrane foot process fusion (5).

2. *Differential Diagnostic Procedures*

a) Estimate of kidney size and configuration, evidence of obstruction: flat plate of abdomen, renal ultrasound, intravenous pyelogram. These tests are listed from the least to the most invasive. If reliable and complete information is obtained with the least invasive, it is usually not necessary to proceed to the more invasive procedure. Renal arteriography is usually not necessary, but venography may be performed to rule out renal vein thrombosis. Some radiologists feel that paying careful attention to the venous phase of renal angiography is a better way to diagnose renal vein thrombosis than venography.

b) Search for systemic causes: includes blood and urine tests to rule out the occurrence of the nephrotic syndrome in the setting of, or associated with, systemic disease. This would include serologic tests for lupus, blood sugar (and perhaps glucose tolerance test) to uncover diabetic nephropathy, serum protein electrophoresis to diagnose multiple myloma, etc. (see Table 2-1 for etiologic categories).

c) Search for evidence of immunologically mediated renal disease: This includes determinations of serum complement levels (especially C_3 and C_4), C_3 nephritic factor and anti-glomerular basement membrane antibodies (where indicated), evidence of circulating immune complexes and evidence for recent infection (antistreptolysin and antihyaluronidase titers, hepatitis antigen, etc.).

d) Renal biopsy. It has been the custom of the author and his colleagues to biopsy most patients with nephrotic syndrome before beginning a treatment regimen. Exceptions to this include 1) patients in whom the diagnosis of diabetic nephropathy has been made and there are no atypical features of the patient's illness. If the presentation is atypical, we would probably biopsy if renal function is reasonably well preserved; 2) patients who have had a biopsy prior to the development of the nephrotic

TABLE 2-1. Etiologic Categories of Nephrotic Syndrome[a]

A. Post infectious
   1. Bacterial—streptococcus, staphylococcus, syphilis, tuberculosis
   2. Viral—hepatitis B, CMV, EBV, herpes, varicella
   3. Protozoal—toxoplasma, malaria
   4. Helminthic—filiaria, schistosoma, trypanosoma

B. Drugs
   Gold, mercury, heroin, penicillamine, probenecid, etc.

C. Neoplasms
   Solid tumors, lymphoma and leukemia

D. "Connective Tissue" Diseases
   Systemic lupus erythematosis, polyarteritis, Sjögren's syndrome

E. Other Multisystem Disorders
   Amyloidosis, diabetes mellitus, Goodpasture's syndrome, Henoch-Schöenlein purpura, myxedema, sarcoidosis, etc.

F. Allergic Reactions
   Bee sting, pollens, poison ivy, etc.

G. Inherited Disorders
   Alport's syndrome, familial nephrotic syndrome, Fabry's disease, etc.

H. Miscellaneous
   Malignant hypertension, constrictive pericarditis, pre-eclampsia, etc.

I. Idiopathic Nephrotic Syndrome (See Table 2-3)

[a]For more complete compilations of etiopathogenetic considerations, the reader is referred to references 7 and 8.

syndrome and in whom there are no clinical features to suggest that a different disease process is now present; and 3) patients who decline renal biopsy or in whom it is contraindicated (bleeding abnormality, solitary kidney).

Treatment

1. General Measures

a) Bed rest and sodium restriction may suffice in patients with mild to moderate edema, especially if they have never been treated for nephrotic edema before.

b) Hypoalbuminemia may be helped by encouraging the patient to eat a diet that contains high-biologic-value protein. Dietary manipulation of this kind will be limited if the patient has substantial renal insufficiency or renal failure, in which case protein may need to be restricted.

2. *Therapy of the Underlying Disease Process*

The reader is directed again to the list of etiologic factors provided in Table 2-1. A perusal of this extensive catalogue of diagnostic possibilities will provide information as to obvious therapeutic measures. This would include, for example, the withdrawal of potentially offending drugs; a search for and treatment of solid tumors and lymphoproliferative disorders; the elimination of infection; and investigation and treatment of so-called connective tissue diseases (7, 8). In a significant proportion of patients, a diagnosis of idiopathic nephrotic syndrome will be made (7). In this group, renal biopsy will be helpful, along with the clinical history, in determining whether immunosuppressive therapy will be helpful or not (Table 2-2).

In Table 2-3 the various potential etiologies of nephrotic syndrome are categorized according to their response to treatment. When treatment is undertaken, prednisone is the most frequently employed drug, in a dosage of 60–80 mg per day or 120–150 mg every other day. Cyclophosphamide and azathioprine have also been utilized, separately or in combination with steroids (7, 8). Cyclophosphamide may be employed alone in Wegener's granulomatosis. It should be recognized that the majority of the observations on this topic are the result of uncontrolled studies and anecdotal experience.

3. *Diuretic Therapy*

Diuretics are often useful in the following categories of patients: 1) in those patients who have not responded to salt restriction and bed rest; 2) in patients who need their edema controlled while a therapeutic trial of immunosuppressive agents is attempted; 3) in those patients who have failed immunosuppressive therapy; and 4) in those patients in whom no specific therapy (immunosuppressive or otherwise) is considered effective for their particular lesions.

Specific diuretic regimens are given in Table 2-4. As noted above, when one is dealing with mild disease, bed rest and sodium restriction may suffice. This is especially true when the immunosuppressive or other therapy has been started and one is awaiting a remission of the patient's disease process. However, steroids can cause sodium retention and may make the edema worse.

Should mild edema not respond to these simple measures, then drugs of the thiazide group or metolazone may be started. In keeping with the general principles of diuretic therapy (see Chapter 1), the mildest agent which will accomplish the therapeutic purpose should be employed. Only if the edema is moderate to severe, or if it does not respond to the agents listed above, should therapy with the drugs that primarily inhibit transport in the ascending limb of the loop of Henle be employed. Unlike the

TABLE 2-2. Idiopathic Nephrotic Syndrome: Histologic Classification and Significance of the Lesion

A. Minimal change disease ("nil" disease, "lipoid nephrosis")
   1. Light microscopy shows little if any abnormality. Electron microscopy reveals fusion of the foot processes (podocytes) of the glomerular basement membrane.
   2. May spontaneously remit (especially in children); usually responds well to steroid therapy.

B. Proliferative glomerulonephritis
   1. Light microscopy shows an increase in cells in the glomeruli, which can originate from the epithelium, the endothelium or can represent leukocytes, or any combination of these. Immunofluorescence studies of the glomeruli may show the presence of immunoglobulin and/or complement.
   2. May respond to steroids or steroids plus cytotoxic therapy; a large group of non-responders does exist, however.

C. Membranous glomerulonephritis
   1. Light microscopy shows thickened glomerular basement membrane (GBM); in advanced disease, splitting and disorganization of the GBM may be evident. Electron microscopy confirms the light microscopic picture and often demonstrates the presence of electron-dense deposits, usually subepithelial in position.
   2. Spontaneous remission reported in a minority of patients; the matter of response to immunosuppressive therapy is controversial; recent studies suggest steroids may be helpful, cytotoxic drugs probably are not.

D. Membranoproliferative glomerulonephritis ("mesangiocapillary" glomerulonephritis)
   1. Occurs in two types
      a. Type I—mesangial cell proliferation associated with thickening of the GBM; there may be subendothelial deposits.
      b. Type II—in addition to proliferative features, intramembranous deposits are present ("dense deposit disease").
   2. Frequently is associated with persistent hypocomplementemia.
   3. Spontaneous remission is unusual; type I may respond to immunosuppressive therapy but type II probably does not.

E. Focal glomerulosclerosis ("focal sclerosis")
   1. Patchy involvement of glomeruli with sclerotic lesions; not all of the glomeruli are affected, and in those in which the process is present, usually only a portion of the individual glomerulus is involved.
   2. Usually this lesion does not respond either to steroids or cytotoxic agents.

thiazides, and especially metolazone and chlorthalidone, which may have effects lasting for 24 hr, the "loop blockers" are usually not effective for more than 4–6 hr and, therefore, may have to be given more than once a day.

In cases of severe edema, it may be necessary to blockade sodium reabsorption at more than one site in the nephron (see Chapter 1). A rather potent combination, in the author's experience, is that of metolazone and a loop diuretic (see Table 2-3). Patients with resistant edema, as

TABLE 2-3. Immunosuppressive Therapy in the Nephrotic Syndrome

A. Immunosuppressive therapy probably beneficial
   1. minimal change glomerulonephritis ("nil" disease, "lipoid nephrosis")
   2. membranous glomerulonephritis[a]
   3. lupus nephritis[b]
   4. polyarteritis nodosa
   5. Wegener's granulomatosis[c]
   6. Sjögren's syndrome

B. Immunosuppressive therapy possibly beneficial
   1. membranoproliferative glomerulonephritis, type I
   2. Henoch-Schoenlein purpura
   3. Goodpasture's syndrome[d]

C. Immunosuppressive therapy probably not helpful
   1. proliferative glomerulonephritis
   2. focal glomerular sclerosis
   3. membranoproliferative glomerulonephritis, type II (dense deposit disease)

D. Immunosuppressive therapy not indicated (or contraindicated) for treatment of nephrotic syndrome
   1. multiple myeloma
   2. amyloidosis
   3. neoplasms (except lymphoma, where "immunosuppressive" therapy of the primary disease may lead to a remission of the nephrotic syndrome)
   4. hereditary nephritis
   5. diabetic nephropathy

[a]Steroid therapy probably of no benefit in advanced disease with severe glomerular basement membrane changes and/or markedly reduced renal function.
[b]Immunosuppressive therapy may not be helpful in some forms of lupus nephritis (e.g., the diffuse proliferative variety).
[c]Cyclophosphamide therapy (usually without steroids) is usually recommended.
[d]Plasmapheresis may be beneficial either alone or combined with immunosuppressive therapy.

characterized by failure to respond to oral combination therapy as outpatients, should be hospitalized. Not only does admission guarantee compliance with medication, but it provides some assurance that bed rest and low sodium intake can be accomplished. If it is not clear that the patient has been taking his/her diuretics as an out-patient, hospitalizing the patient and instituting the combination therapy he/she was supposedly taking as an out-patient, may suffice. If there is no response, then one should move to intravenous therapy as outlined in Table 2-3 (section D). As discussed under General Guidelines in Chapter 1, when switching from oral to intravenous drug, the dose should be lowered. Oral metolazone plus IV furosemide has been an effective regimen in our experience. Failure with gradually increasing doses of drug should prompt

TABLE 2-4. Sample Diuretic Regimens for the Therapy of the Nephrotic Syndrome

A. Mild edema (not responsive to bed rest and/or sodium restriction)
   1. Hydrochlorothiazide, 25–100 mg administered p.o. daily (usually in the morning), or every other day, or five days out of seven; or
   2. Metolazone, 2.5–5 mg, administered by the same general schedule as for hydrochlorothiazide.

B. Moderate edema (especially if not responsive to therapies listed in A)
   1. Furosemide, 40–120′ mg given orally in the morning, with repeat dose later in the day, prn.
   2. Ethacrynic acid, 50–150 mg, administered orally according to the schedule in 1 (above).
   3. Bumetanide, 1–3 mg orally, on a schedule similar to that for furosemide or ethacrynic acid.

C. Severe edema
   1. Metolazone 5–10 mg p.o. every morning combined with furosemide 80–160 mg as a single oral dose in the morning. If diuresis occurs but does not reach the magnitude required to satisfy the therapeutic goal, the furosemide may be repeated later in the day; or
   2. Hydrochlorothiazide, 50–100 mg orally in the morning, combined with furosemide (see C 1, above), or bumetanide, 1–3 mg, or ethacrynic acid 50–200 mg as a single dose, given orally.

D. "Resistant" edema
   1. Hospitalize the patient, place at bed rest and begin on 2 gm Na^+ diet.
   2. Switch from oral to IV drug, e.g.,
      a. begin with 40 mg of furosemide or 50 mg of ethacrynic acid or 1 mg of bumetanide.
      b. If no response, add oral metolazone 5–10 mg or hydrochlorothiazide 50–100 mg (oral or IV) to the loop blockade. If oral drug is being given, wait one hr before injecting furosemide, ethacrynic acid or bumetanide IV.
      c. If no response in 2–3 hr, administer double dose of the loop diuretic. If the patient responds, dose may be repeated in 6–12 hr if indicated. Daily IV drug may be given until clinical circumstances suggest that a return to oral therapy is appropriate (reduction in or disappearance of edema, improvement in GFR, etc).
      d. If no response, continue oral metolazone (or hydrochlorothiazide), give intravenous loop diuretic and add intravenous albumin, 12.5–25.0 gm infused over 2–3 hr. The loop diuretic and albumin may be repeated later in the day, if necessary, but there is no reason to repeat metolazone, which is long-acting.
   3. It may be worthwhile to add a "potassium-sparing" agent. An example of such a regimen: 5–10 mg metolazone in the morning, 25–50 mg of spironolactone QID, and 120 mg of furosemide IV one hr after the p.o. metolazone. The thiazides may be given instead of metolazone and triamterene 50–100 mg BID or amiloride 5–10 mg daily can replace the spironolactone.
   4. Patients who do not respond to combination diuretic therapy plus albumin infusion generally require dialysis. The latter is rarely necessary if GFR is above 10–15 ml/min.

the addition of albumin infusion to the regimen. Patients who do not respond to these therapeutic maneuvers will require dialysis.

Overvigorous therapy and massive natriuresis are to be avoided. The incidence of the side effects of the diuretics (especially "loop" drugs) is increased by giving very large doses (a practice we do not recommend) and by giving the drugs intravenously (see Chapter 11). Finally, replacement of potassium or addition of a "potassium-sparing" diuretic will often be required. The latter group of drugs is usually employed for one or both of the following two reasons: 1) to blockade sodium transport at as many sites in the nephron as possible in association with the use of two other agents (see Chapter 1), and 2) to minimize the kaliuresis which will accompany the natriuresis associated with the use of potent diuretic agents.

References

1. Bernard, D.B., Alexander, E.A., Couser, W.G., and Levinsky, N.F. Renal sodium retention during volume expansion in experimental nephrotic syndrome. Kidney Int. 14:478–485, 1978.
2. Ichikawa, I., Rennke, H.G., Hoyer, J.R., Badr, K.F., Schor, N., Troy, J.L., Lechene, C.P., and Brenner, B.M. Role for intrarenal mechanisms in the impaired salt excretion of experimental nephrotic syndrome. J. Clin. Invest. 71:91–103, 1983.
3. Grausz, H., Lieberman, R., and Earley, L.E. Effect of plasma albumin on sodium reabsorption in patients with nephrotic syndrome. Kidney Int. 1:47–54, 1972.
4. Kassirer, J.P., and Gennari, F.J. Laboratory evaluation of renal function. In: Strauss and Welt's Diseases of the Kidney, 3rd edition, 1979 (editors: L.E. Earley and C.W. Gottschalk), Boston, Little Brown and Co., pp. 41–92.
5. Brezin, J.H., Katz, S.M., Schwartz, A.B., Chinitz, J.L. Reversible renal failure and nephrotic syndrome associated with nonsteroidal antiinflammatory drugs. N. Engl. J. Med. 23:1271–1273, 1979.
6. Gary, N.E., Dodelson, R., and Eisinger, R.P. Indomethacin-associated acute renal failure. Am. J. Med. 69:135–136, 1980.
7. Glassock, R.J., Cohen, A.H., Bennett, C.M., and Martinez-Maldonado, M. Primary glomerular diseases. In: The Kidney, 2nd edition, 1981 (editors: B.M. Brenner and F.C. Rector, Jr.), Philadelphia, W.B. Saunders Co., pp. 1351–1492.
8. Earley, L.E., and Forland, M. Nephrotic syndrome. In: Strauss and Welt's Diseases of the Kidney, 3rd edition, 1979 (editors: L.E. Earley and C.W. Gottschalk), Boston, Little Brown and Co., pp. 765–813.

chapter

3

Diuretic Therapy in the Patient with Edema/Ascites Associated with Hepatic Disease

Arthur Greenberg, M.D.

Ascites and edema, the cardinal findings of hepatic cirrhosis, are accompanied by avid renal sodium retention. The accumulation of ascites and edema is an important cause of morbidity and much patient and physician effort is devoted to their elimination. As with other disorders of sodium retention, dietary salt restriction and diuretics are the principal means of control. Complications of overvigorous diuresis include volume depletion, hypokalemia with worsened hepatic encephalopathy, and renal failure and death due to the hepatorenal syndrome. To reduce the risk of such problems, diuretic use should be parsimonious and the physician and patient should remain conservative in their goals.

Pathogenesis of Sodium Retention in Cirrhosis

Two theories have been promoted to explain the renal sodium retention seen in hepatic cirrhosis. According to the classic "underfilling" theory (Figure 3-1, panel A), the primary lesion resides in the liver. Altered hepatic sinusoidal architecture with increased intrahepatic hydrostatic pressure from portal hypertension leads to transudation of ascites from the liver into the peritoneal cavity in an amount in excess of that which can be removed by the lymphatics. In addition, hypoalbuminemia due to impaired hepatic albumin synthesis alters the capillary Starling forces in such a way as to favor the transudation of fluid into the abdominal cavity from the liver and mesenteric lymphatics and into dependent tissue interstitial spaces as edema. This loss of fluid leads to a decrease in intravascular volume. The kidney attempts to compensate by retaining sodium and fluid.

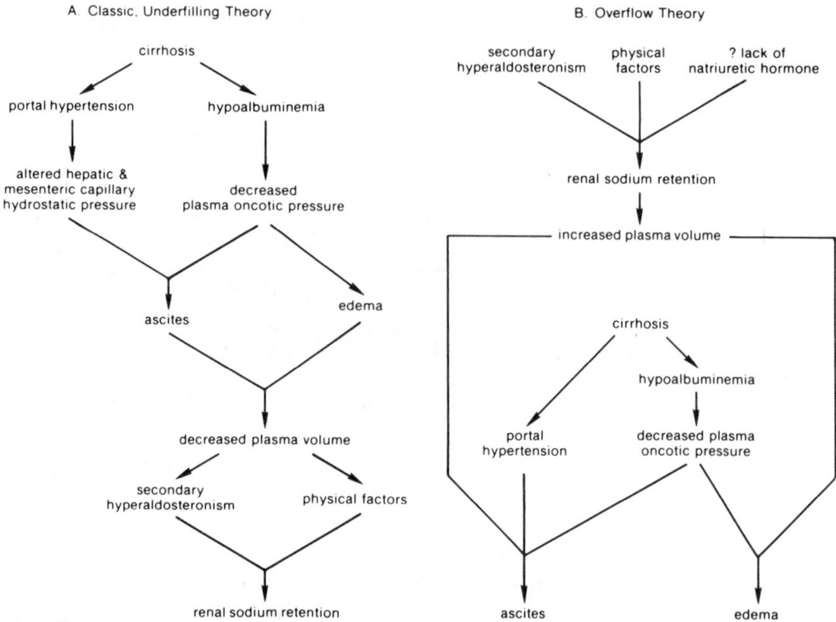

Figure 3-1. Pathogenesis of sodium retention in cirrhosis.

The mechanisms for renal compensation are several. Renin, angiotensin, and aldosterone levels are known to be increased in cirrhosis. The increase in aldosterone leads to increased sodium reabsorption by the distal nephron. In the proximal nephron, renal sodium reabsorption is also increased. The determinants of proximal nephron sodium reabsorption are incompletely understood. They are known to include physical forces related to glomerular arteriolar vasoconstriction with decreased post glomerular capillary hydrostatic pressure and altered filtration fraction with a resultant increase in post-glomerular capillary oncotic pressure. In addition, the existence of a "third factor," a natriuretic hormone acting in the proximal nephron, has been postulated but not proven. An additional cause of renal sodium retention may be decreased GFR with decreased filtered load of sodium.

The alternative explanation for the sodium retention seen in cirrhosis is the "overflow" theory as promoted by Lieberman (1). Here, sodium retention occurs because the hormonal or physical factors detailed above are somehow stimulated directly by liver disease without a prior decrease in intravascular volume. According to this hypothesis, renal sodium retention is the primary event leading to ascites and edema formation. Because of the altered hepatic capillary bed, the retained salt and water leak into the abdominal cavity as ascites. In addition, because of hypoalbuminemia, the excess salt and fluid spill into the interstitium as edema. This proposal is illustrated in panel B of Figure 3-1.

A large body of experimental data has been amassed favoring one or the other alternative (2). It is clear that available measurements indicate that plasma volume is either normal or increased rather than decreased in cirrhosis. Also, in a series of studies on dogs with experimentally induced cirrhosis, Levy has shown that renal sodium retention precedes ascites formation and that ascites and edema formation can be prevented if sodium restriction is instituted early, while cirrhosis is still developing (3). These two lines of evidence seem to favor the overflow theory.

Support for the classic theory includes the findings in several studies that rapid volume repletion with colloid or saline solutions or restoration of central volume by head-out water immersion can lead to a diuresis. Furthermore, in cirrhotics, vasopressin and norepinephrine levels are increased. As levels of these hormones are known to increase as part of the compensatory mechanism for hemorrhage and true volume depletion, the increase in their blood levels suggests that the body and the kidney are behaving as though the plasma volume were decreased. Taken at face value, these findings contradict the experimental data showing an increased plasma volume in cirrhosis. Proponents of the underfilling theory maintain that it is the unmeasurable but important "effective plasma volume" that is decreased in cirrhosis and discount the importance of the direct plasma volume measurements. It must also be noted that the proposed mechanism for the sodium retention in the overflow theory, the failure of a diseased liver to make a natriuretic hormone or to detoxify a sodium retentive substance, has not yet been confirmed by isolation of such substances from normal or pathologic subjects or experimental animals. The assumption that one of these rather simple formulations explains the many defects seen in cirrhosis is undoubtedly an oversimplification.

Obviously, cirrhotics are not all alike. At one end of the spectrum are those patients who have well-preserved renal function and a tendency to edema and ascites formation. At the other end are patients with the hepatorenal syndrome. Simply defined, this disorder is the development of irreversible oliguric renal failure associated with marked sodium retention in the setting of far advanced hepatic cirrhosis (4). By definition, other causes of renal failure such as acute tubular necrosis due to hypotension after a variceal bleed or due to administration of nephrotoxic drugs are excluded. The disorder may develop insidiously or abruptly. In a series of elegant and heroic studies, Tristani and Cohn studied a large group of such patients and found that they could be subdivided into two groups on the basis of cardiac index (5). The group with lower cardiac index behaved as though cirrhosis and ascites had developed according to the underfilling theory. They had lower plasma volumes, cardiac outputs, and renal blood flow and higher peripheral and renal vascular resistances. They responded to volume repletion with dextran by increasing cardiac output and renal blood flow and by decreasing total peripheral vascular resistance. The patients in the other group had higher cardiac indexes and behaved as though they were volume expanded. Total peripheral vascular resistances were low and little response was seen to expansion. The hemodynamic parameters in this group resembled those to be expected in the presence of a large arteriovenous shunt.

The Rationale for Cautious Treatment of Ascites and Edema

In few other conditions than cirrhosis must the physician be more mindful of the dictum, *primum non nocere*. Treatment of cirrhotic edema is fraught with complications. Resolution of ascites and edema is seldom an emergency. Ascites and edema take a long time to accumulate and should be allowed a long time to resolve. The only instance where there is any urgency is where ascites contributes to respiratory embarrassment. Here, judicious paracentesis with removal of only a liter of fluid should ameliorate respiratory distress. This will allow time for formulation of a plan for gradual diuresis.

Diuretics act by decreasing renal sodium reabsorption and promoting excretion of salt and water already contained within the intravascular space. They do not act on ascitic fluid or edema fluid directly. The ascites and edema respond to diuretic treatment because diuretic-induced loss of salt and water lowers intravascular hydrostatic pressure enough so that Starling forces favor absorption of ascitic and edema fluid back into the intravascular space. Shear and Gabuzda have shown that the maximum rate of ascites reabsorption is approximately 900 ml per day (6). Edema fluid can be reabsorbed somewhat more rapidly. In a patient with ascites alone, it is clear that attempts to promote a net diuresis of more than 1 liter per day are extremely likely to induce intravascular volume depletion. Induction of volume depletion tends to stimulate proximal sodium avidity and to increase production of aldosterone with consequent stimulation of distal sodium reabsorption. These two effects make further diuresis more difficult. It also bears emphasis that volume depletion leads to tissue hypoperfusion, a condition clearly not beneficial to the patient, and is a risk factor for the development of irreversible hepatorenal syndrome.

A second major diuretic complication is hypokalemia. Because of chronic hyperaldosteronism, cirrhotic patients typically have a modest total body potassium deficit. Because of high circulating levels of aldosterone, their kidneys are prepared to excrete large amounts of potassium in exchange for sodium. Administration of diuretics which increase delivery of sodium to the distal nephron sodium-potassium-hydrogen exchange site (see Figure 1-2) is likely to cause a marked

TABLE 3-1. Suggested Diuretic Regimen for Therapy of Cirrhosis with Ascites and Edema

1. *Goal*
   ½–1 kg/day weight loss if both ascites and edema present; ½ kg/day if ascites present alone
2. *General measures*
   Bedrest, daily weights, intake and output measurements; BUN, creatinine, electrolytes at least on alternate days
3. *Diet*
   20–40 meq sodium (500–1000 mg sodium); liberalize only if diuresis is successful
4. *Diuretics*
   Add sequentially:
   Spironolactone 100 mg in divided doses; increase to 400 mg daily
   Hydrochlorothiazide 50 mg; give up to 100 mg daily
   Furosemide 40 mg p.o. starting dose; increase to 240 mg b.i.d.
5. Diuretic resistance
   a. If above regimen fails:
      Check 24–hr sodium excretion on above regimen.
      If high, adjust diet
      If low, continue spironolactone and
      Begin furosemide 40 mg IV, increase dose to 240 mg IV b.i.d.
   b. If this fails, add sequentially:
      Metolazone 5–20 mg p.o. (as single a.m. dose);
      Salt poor albumin 25–50 mg IV before furosemide

kaliuresis and lead to hypokalemia or exacerbate established hypokalemia. Renal ammoniogenesis is a function of blood potassium concentration. Hypokalemia augments renal ammonia production. This does not cause a problem in normal subjects who become hypokalemic, but cirrhotics with marginal hepatic function are unable to handle the increased ammonia load. Thus, the induction of hypokalemia with diuretics may lead to the development of or worsening of hepatic encephalopathy.

There are several other potential diuretic complications. Although spironolactone is frequently used to obviate hypokalemia, its use is not without side effects. Spironolactone has been shown not only to antagonize potassium exchange for sodium but also to diminish hydrogen ion exchange for sodium in the distal nephron. This effect is of minor importance in normal subjects but in cirrhotics, administration of spironolactone can lead to hyperkalemic metabolic acidosis (7). Administration of the kaliuretic diuretics, by contrast, is associated with augmented hydrogen ion loss and development of metabolic alkalosis. Diuretic use may also contribute to the development of hyponatremia. For several reasons, cirrhotics are already at risk for hyponatremia. First, basal vasopressin levels are increased. Second, because of proximal nephron sodium avidity, delivery of salt and water to the distal diluting sites may be reduced. These two factors combine to decrease the renal ability to excrete free water. Furthermore, when distal delivery is further reduced and the volume stimulus to vasopressin release is further augmented by diuretic induced volume depletion, the ability to excrete free water will be more severely impaired. In addition, diuretics like furosemide and the thiazides that act at the diluting sites impair free water generation by yet another mechanism. It is clear from studies by Sherlock and others that the incidence of diuretic-induced complications is related to the nature and potency of the diuretic used (8). This is due not only to factors inherent to the diuretics but is also due to the need to use a more complicated diuretic regimen in patients with more severe hepatic disease.

Therapy of Cirrhotic Ascites and Edema

The treatment of cirrhotics requires careful planning and, above all, patience. The therapeutic regimen should begin with simple measures and additional maneuvers or diuretics should be added in stepwise fashion only when earlier measures have proved inadequate. Sufficient time must be allowed for response to any maneuver before a new one is added. Such a plan will minimize the complications of diuretic treatment. This therapeutic approach has been demonstrated to be successful (9).

1. *Goals*

In achieving a diuresis the aim is, of course, to cause sodium and water excretion to exceed sodium and water intake. The lower the intake the smaller the excretion need be to achieve negative balance. Because of the risk of hepatorenal syndrome and the electrolyte abnormalities enumerated above, the diuresis must be designed to proceed at a slow pace. Although edema can be mobilized more rapidly, the maximum rate of ascites mobilization is 900 ml per day. Thus, the rate of fluid removal should be moderate. A kilogram per day may be removed safely in patients with edema and ascites but a reasonable goal for patients with ascites alone is 0.5 kg per day. If the weight loss is occurring at a more rapid rate, then therapy should be modified to slow the rate.

2. *General Measures*

As with any patient with edema, careful monitoring is necessary to assess a response to therapy. Routine orders should include daily weight determinations as well as careful intake and output measurements and frequent electrolyte, BUN, and serum creatinine determinations.

3. *Diet*

The dietary sodium should be severely restricted. A reasonable starting diet is one containing 20–40 meq, or approximately 500–1000 mg of sodium per day. This is not a palatable diet which a patient can follow at home but it can be achieved for the short term in the hospital. The patient and his family should be cautioned about supplementing this hospital diet with food brought from the outside. The physician must himself be meticulous about administration of salt with intravenous fluids. Recall that each liter of 0.9% saline contains 154 meq of sodium and even 0.2% saline contains 34 meq (787 mg) of sodium per liter. If the diuresis proceeds satisfactorily, the salt intake may be liberalized. Water restriction is not necessary unless hyponatremia develops.

4. *Diuretic Therapy*

Sodium restriction alone is adequate to induce a diuresis in 10–15% of patients. Three to four days should be allowed to assess the response to sodium restriction alone and, ideally, three to four days should elapse between each stepwise addition of or increase in diuretics. The author recognizes that time constraints do not allow for such a conservative approach in all instances.

The diuretic to be begun initially is spironolactone. This drug is a competitive inhibitor of aldosterone and has the dual advantages of being antikaliuretic and of having only a modest natriuretic effect (see also Chapter 1 and Appendix 2). As such, spironolactone alone is unlikely to lead to an overrapid diuresis or to cause hypokalemia. It should be begun as 100 mg daily in two to four divided doses and the dosage gradually increased. Most patients destined to respond will do so to a dose of 200 mg daily although a few will require 400 mg. At least 48 hr is required to assess the effect of a given daily dosage of this agent. Some investigators find it useful to follow the urine sodium:potassium ratio during spironolactone treatment (10). A urine sodium:potassium ratio less than 1 suggests persistence of aldosterone effect. A ratio greater than 1 suggests that aldosterone effect is fully blocked. In the author's experience, this ratio has not been terribly useful since the diuretic response is really best judged by following the patient's weight. Serial measurement of urine sodium excretion can, however, emphasize the marked avidity seen with cirrhosis, as the kidney can achieve urine sodium concentrations less than 1 meq per day with excretion of a urine virtually free of sodium. Approximately 40–60% of patients will respond to dietary sodium restriction and spironolactone.

If no diuresis has resulted after the maximum dosage of spironolactone has been reached, then more potent diuretics should be added. Hydrochlorothiazide can be begun at a dose of 50 mg per day and increased to a total dose of 100 mg per day. If hydrochlorothiazide does not induce a diuresis, a loop diuretic should be prescribed. Furosemide 40 mg daily should be begun as a single dose. If no response is seen to 40 mg of furosemide, its dose may be increased in 40 mg increments. Furosemide works best when given in one or two large doses daily. Although there is no fixed upper limit to the daily dosage of furosemide, little additional benefit is seen with an increase in dose above 240 mg p.o. twice daily.

5. *Refractory Edema*

Diuretic refractoriness, defined as the failure of a reasonable dose of a loop diuretic to induce a diuresis, is not an uncommon occurrence in cirrhosis. In general, there are several potential causes for diuretic refractoriness. To be effective, a diuretic must reach its site of action in the nephron and it must inhibit sodium or chloride reabsorption at that site. Diuretics may fail to reach their site of action because of administration error or patient noncompliance. In addition, orally administered agents will fail if bowel wall edema reduces absorption and bioavailability. True diuretic resistance occurs if the stimuli promoting sodium or chloride reabsorption at the diuretic site in question are abnormally strong or augmented reabsorption at more proximal sites has substantially reduced the amount of fluid reaching the site where the diuretic acts. Similarly, diuretics fail if sodium delivery to the tubular lumen is reduced by a fall in filtered load due to low GFR.

In trying to decide why a patient has not lost weight despite what seems to be an appropriate diuretic regimen, two questions must be asked. First, has the drug been given as ordered? Medication records should be reviewed. Second, is the patient really failing to excrete sodium in response to the diuretic? Measurement of 24-hr urine sodium excretion in an attempt to measure sodium balance is helpful in this determination. It is clear that a diuresis occurs only if salt excretion exceeds salt intake. As the electrolyte composition of edema fluid is similar to that of plasma, excretion of approximately 140 meq of sodium is required to achieve a loss of 1 kg of edema fluid. Not infrequently, a diuretic is successful in promoting sodium excretion but a diuresis fails to occur because the patient's sodium intake is much higher than that prescribed. If the measured daily sodium excretion is high but the weight is stable, then the physician can infer that the sodium intake is also high. For example, if a patient is excreting in excess of 100 meq of sodium each day but his weight has remained constant, then his dietary intake must also be on the order of 100 meq. Reduction in sodium intake in such a patient would lead to a prompt weight loss.

The direct measurement of oral drug absorption is impractical. If sodium excretion has not increased in response to large doses of oral diuretics, the next step is to switch the route of administration to IV. Intravenous furosemide, in doses of up to 240 mg twice daily, should be tried. As intravenous administration bypasses the intestine, failure to respond to IV furosemide is indicative of true diuretic refractoriness. The physician should then attempt sequential blockade of all nephron sodium reabsorption sites. The addition of metolazone, in a single daily dose of up to 20 mg to the regimen already including spironolactone and furosemide, is a useful one in the author's experience. With cirrhotic edema, two additional methods of removal of ascites are available. First, hyperoncotic albumin may be administered. Acutely, this favors the mobilization of fluid back into the intravascular space from which its excretion may be stimulated by maximal doses of diuretics. A regimen incorporating albumin would include 400 mg of spironolactone in divided doses along with 20 mg of metolazone followed in 30 minutes by 25 gm of salt poor albumin and 240 mg of IV furosemide. In rare cases, a response will be seen to 400 mg of IV furosemide. Doses this high should be infused over an hour to minimize ototoxicity.

If all of these measures have failed, then a mechanical diversion procedure such as the LeVeen peritoneovenous shunt may be considered. This procedure is not without risk of major complication, including disseminated intravascular coagulation, pyrogenic reactions and sepsis, and it should be considered only in patients who have failed all conservative measures. Its use is best reserved for centers which have accumulated a large experience with this procedure.

6. *Treatment of Complications*

The treatment of complications such as hypokalemia, hyperkalemia, metabolic acidosis, or metabolic alkalosis is self-evident and deserves only brief mention. If spironolactone treatment has led to hyperkalemia and metabolic acidosis, the drug should be stopped and then resumed later in a lower dosage. Hypokalemia and metabolic alkalosis due to hydrochlorothiazide or furosemide should be treated with potassium supplementation. It may also be necessary to stop the drugs for a brief period. Alternatively, spironolactone may be added or its dosage increased if it is already being employed. Potassium supplements should not be used in patients receiving spironolactone, as refractory hyperkalemia can be produced rather easily.

Azotemia is the most dreaded diuretic complication. Cirrhotic patients tread a thin line between ascites and edema on the one side and intravascular volume depletion on the other. It is impossible to distinguish clinically between prerenal azotemia due to diuretic use and the hepatorenal syndrome. If azotemia develops in the course of diuretic therapy, the diuretics should be stopped and albumin begun in an effort to expand the intravascular space. Once azotemia has resolved, the diuretics may be cautiously resumed in lower dose. The physician is wise to be satisfied with incomplete resolution of edema and ascites in this setting.

References

1. Lieberman, F.L., Denison, E.K., and Reynolds, T.B. The relationship of plasma volume, portal hypertension, ascites and renal sodium retention in cirrhosis: The overflow theory of ascites formation. Ann. NY Acad. Sci. 170:202–206, 1970.
2. Epstein, M. Deranged sodium homeostasis in cirrhosis. Gastroenterology 76:622–635, 1979.
3. Levy, M. Observations on renal function and ascites formation in dogs with experimental portal cirrhosis. In: The Kidney in Liver Disease, 1978 (editor: M. Epstein). New York, Elsevier North-Holland, pp. 131–142.
4. Conn, H.O. A rational approach to the hepatorenal syndrome. Gastroenterology 65:321–340, 1973.
5. Tristani, F.E., and Cohn, J.N. Systemic and renal hemodynamics in oliguric hepatic failure: effect of volume expansion. J. Clin. Invest. 46:1894–1906, 1967.
6. Shear, L., Ching, S., and Gabuzda, G.J. Compartmentalization of ascites and edema in patients with hepatic cirrhosis. N. Engl. J. Med. 282:1391–1396, 1970.
7. Gabow, P.A., Moore, S., and Schrier, R.W. Spironolactone-induced hyperchloremic acidosis in cirrhosis. Ann. Int. Med. 90:338–340, 1979.
8. Sherlock, S., Senewiratne, B., Scott, A., and Walker, J.G. Complications of diuretic therapy in hepatic cirrhosis. Lancet 1:1049–1053, 1966.
9. Gregory, P.G., Broekelschen, P.H., Hill, M.D., Lipton, A.B., Knauer, C.M., Egger, J., and Miller, R. Complications of diuresis in the alcoholic patient with ascites: a controlled trial. Gastroenterology 73:534–538, 1977.
10. Eggert, R.C. Spironolactone diuresis in patients with cirrhosis and ascites. Brit. Med. J. 4:401–403, 1970.

chapter

4

Diuretics in the Treatment of Congestive Heart Failure

Arthur Greenberg, M.D.

When cardiac output is insufficient to provide adequate perfusion, heart failure is diagnosed. Sodium retention by the kidney is one of the compensatory mechanisms involved in correction of this disorder. The treatment of congestive failure includes measures to improve cardiac output primarily and to alleviate the vasoconstriction, increased venous pressure, and fluid retention which have been produced in compensation. Diuretics are an important part of the physician's treatment armamentarium. The choice of agent and its dosage and route of administration vary with the severity of congestive failure and the speed of correction required.

The Mechanism of Sodium Retention in Congestive Heart Failure

The onset of congestive heart failure is heralded by a fall in arterial distending pressure. The earliest response to this decrease in "effective arterial volume" is an increase in sympathetic tone. This acts to restore cardiac output by several means. Catecholamines have a direct inotropic and chronotropic effect on the heart and increase cardiac output by increasing both force of contractility and heart rate. In addition, catecholamines lead to vasoconstriction. Venoconstriction decreases venous pooling and increases venous return and cardiac filling pressures. Arteriolar vasoconstriction directly increases blood pressure and selectively shunts blood to more essential areas. A second hormonal response to the fall in effective arterial volume is an increase in renin secretion and consequently in angiotensin activity. Angiotensin is another potent vasoconstrictor and further contributes to the restoration of blood pressure (1).

The mechanisms enumerated above produce their effects rapidly and are the defense against acute changes in cardiac output. The stimulation of renal sodium retention also occurs at once but only gradually leads to an expansion in total body sodium. In mild to moderate congestive heart failure, the resulting expansion of the extracellular and intravascular space may sufficiently alter venous filling pressures to restore cardiac output to normal. In this case the stimulus for the various compensatory mechanisms is removed and sympathetic tone and renin secretion return to normal. The cost of successful compensation is a modest expansion in total body sodium content. With more severe congestive heart failure, the stimuli remain and sodium retention persists. A sufficiently large increase in intravascular volume leads to an increase in capillary hydrostatic pressure great enough to cause edema.

The mechanisms which allow for renal sodium retention are several and include both proximal and distal factors (2). The augmented distal reabsorption is mediated principally by aldosterone, the release of which is stimulated by renin and angiotensin.

The increase in proximal reabsorption is complex and due mostly to so-called physical factors that shift glomerulotubular balance toward reabsorption. Although renal blood flow falls in parallel with cardiac output, GFR is well preserved in mild to moderate congestive heart failure because the filtration fraction increases. When a greater proportion of fluid is filtered, the oncotic pressure of the fluid remaining behind in the post-glomerular capillaries is higher. This alters Starling forces in such a fashion as to favor sodium and fluid reabsorption. The reduced hydrostatic pressure in the post-glomerular renal capillaries resulting from vasoconstriction induced by increased sympathetic tone also augments reabsorption. Finally, in congestive heart failure, renal blood flow is directed to deeper, juxtamedullary nephrons which seem to be inherently more avid for sodium reabsorption.

With severe congestive heart failure, GFR is decreased with a consequent reduction in sodium excretion. A number of other factors including the lack of a "natriuretic hormone" and renal hemodynamic effects induced by altered prostaglandin synthesis have also been proposed as causes of the abnormal sodium retention. These effects are less well documented.

Treatment of Congestive Heart Failure

The fluid retention resulting from congestive heart failure may be treated in several ways. Digitalis glycosides, catecholamines, and other inotropic agents can be used to increase the force of contraction of the heart.

Vasodilators may be used to alter left and right-sided filling pressures. They augment output of the failing heart by improving run-off or raising filling pressures and improving myocardial length-tension relationships. The emphasis of this chapter, however, will be a discussion of the use of diuretics in directly stimulating renal sodium excretion.

The type of diuretic therapy to be used is determined by the severity of congestive heart failure and the rate at which it must be ameliorated. Patients with pulmonary edema will require immediate treatment with supplemental oxygen, digitalis and intravenous diuretics at the very least. Unloading agents, endotracheal intubation, and catecholamines may be required in selected cases. In contrast, the patient with pedal edema as his only manifestation of congestive heart failure may respond to salt restriction alone. In the severely affected patient, aggressive management should be begun at once. In the patient with mild disease, measures should be begun slowly and additional agents can then be added in stepwise fashion, if needed (3).

1. *Mild Congestive Heart Failure*

Mild congestive heart failure, as evidenced by exertional dyspnea and dependent edema, can often be managed by institution of salt restriction alone. The average American diet may contain in excess of 10 grams per day of sodium. With avoidance of obviously salty foods like potato chips, pretzels, salted nuts, processed meats, and canned soups and elimination of added salt, the diet can easily be reduced to 4 grams per day of sodium. With a few additional proscriptions, the diet can be reduced to 2 grams per day of sodium. With more careful dietary planning, some cooperative patients can follow a 1 gram sodium diet, but this is generally not practicable.

If dietary sodium restriction alone is inadequate, then either a diuretic or digitalis should be added. Digitalis offers the advantage of correcting the underlying problem but the therapeutic margin for digitalis is slim and digitalis toxicity is a frequent complication of therapy. Too much energy has been spent arguing the relative merits of initial treatment with diuretics versus initial treatment with digitalis. This decision is best left to the individual physician based on his assessment of the particular patient. If digitalis alone fails, then a diuretic should be added and vice versa. The diuretic of first choice in this setting is probably furosemide which can be begun as 20–40 mg orally and increased gradually in dose. Hydrochlorothiazide, beginning with a dose of 50 mg daily, may also be used in this setting. It has an additional antihypertensive effect and may be a more suitable starting agent in patients who also have hypertension. In the normotensive patient, furosemide is preferable since thiazide is relatively limited in potency. There is little additional benefit to doses above 100 mg of hydrochlorothiazide daily. Furosemide can be given in doses up to 240 mg twice daily and thus affords a much greater range for titration.

2. *Moderate and Severe Congestive Heart Failure*

Where edema and exertional dyspnea are accompanied by paroxysmal nocturnal dyspnea, orthopnea, or angina, or physical signs including jugular venous distention, rales, or a gallop are present, more aggressive treatment is required. Depending upon the severity of symptoms or the physical findings, it may also be prudent to admit the patient to the hospital at least until initial control is achieved. In this setting both digitalis and furosemide should be used. If not hospitalized, the patient should be given detailed instructions about checking his weight at home daily and reporting back to the physician if symptoms are unimproved and the desired pace of weight loss is not being achieved. For hospitalized patients, the response to diuretic treatment should be monitored carefully with physical exam, input and output measurements and daily weights. As needed, the diuretic dose is increased stepwise. If no response is seen after administration of a given oral dose of furosemide, then twice that dose may be given a few hours later. For example, if 40 mg of furosemide does not lead to a diuresis, 80 mg may be given next and 160 mg after that until the patient begins to respond. Then the dose which has been proven to be effective may be repeated.

TABLE 4-1. Treatment of Congestive Heart Failure

A. Mild or Moderate Congestive Heart Failure
   1. Sodium restriction
   2. Consider hospitalization
   3. Digitalis
   4. Diuretics
      a. Begin with furosemide 20–40 mg po and titrate dose upward
      b. Hydrochlorothiazide 50–100 mg may be useful in hypertensive patients
   5. Monitoring
      a. Check for hypokalemia, metabolic alkalosis, prerenal azotemia
      b. Supplement potassium or add potassium-sparing diuretic as needed

B. Severe (Chronic) Congestive Heart Failure
   1. Sodium restriction
   2. Hospitalize and put at bedrest
   3. Digitalis
   4. Diuretics If regimen described in A-4 (above) has failed:
      a. Begin with furosemide 40 mg IV and titrate dosage upward to 240 mg BID
      b. Use sequential blockade with metolazone, 5–20 mg po and spironolactone 100–400 mg in refractory patients
      c. Reduce doses as pace of diuresis increases with improvement in clinical status

Some patients with severe chronic congestive heart failure will not respond to oral furosemide alone. In these patients, IV furosemide, in a dosage of up to 240 mg BID should be tried next. If this is unsuccessful, sequential blockade (see Chapter 1) with IV furosemide plus metolazone 5–20 mg p.o. as a single dose and spironolactone 100–400 mg p.o. in divided doses should be tried. Spironolactone may lead to gynecomastia; alternatives include triamterene (100–300 mg in divided doses) and amiloride (5–10 mg daily). Caution is required with the antikaliuretic agents as they may lead to severe hyperkalemia in patients with congestive heart failure who may already have a potassium handling defect due to decreased sodium delivery to the distal sodium-potassium exchange sites.

The requirement for diuretics usually decreases as cardiac function improves in response to digitalis or to the salutary effect of the diuresis on filling pressures. The diuretic dose should be reduced accordingly. Obviously, less diuretic will be required to maintain a desired weight than to induce enough diuresis to lead to a net loss of weight. Table 4-1 provides a summary of suggested therapy.

3. *Pulmonary Edema*

With this, the most severe form of left ventricular decompensation, several modalities must be used at once. Supplemental oxygen administration and cardiac monitoring are appropriate in all cases. Morphine, endotracheal intubation, and rotating tourniquets may be required in more severe cases. The diuretic to be used should be a fast-acting, potent diuretic. Furosemide is the standard drug for this situation. It should be given by intravenous route in a starting dose of 40 mg. The time of onset of its diuretic action is 2–10 min. If no response is seen, the drug should be readministered in a dose twice the original dose. This escalation of doses can be continued every 30 min until an effect is seen or a maximum dose of 400 mg has been administered. There is little additional benefit of doses higher than 400 mg. Doses at or above 240 mg should be administered slowly by IV drip because of the risk of ototoxicity. Failure to respond to a dose of this magnitude is usually due to severe congestive heart failure with decreased delivery of fluid to the loop of Henle because of marked proximal nephron sodium avidity or because of an actual decrease in GFR and filtered load. Other means of improving cardiac output, including unloading agents, or potent inotropes like dopamine, dobutamine, or isoproterenol may be necessary. In selected patients, extracorporeal hemofiltration may be considered.

Bumetanide, a recently released loop diuretic, and ethacrynic acid are alternatives to furosemide. Forty milligrams of furosemide, 1 mg of bumetanide and 50 mg of ethacrynic acid are equipotent. Furosemide is

TABLE 4-2. Therapy of Acute Pulmonary Edema

1. Diuretics
   a. Loop diuretics IV as initial therapy.
   b. Begin with furosemide 40 mg (or bumetanide 1 mg) IV. If no effect is seen, serially double the dose until a maximum of 400 mg of furosemide or 5 mg of bumetanide is reached. Use higher starting dose if patient is known to have renal failure.
2. Non-diuretic measures
   Digitalis, supplemental oxygen, monitoring, endotracheal intubation, morphine, and vasodilators, rotating tourniquets, phlebotomy, ultrafiltration.

the preferred agent, except in patients allergic to it, for several reasons. Experience with this agent has shown it to be safe and, like bumetanide, to be much less ototoxic than ethacrynic acid. In addition, furosemide has been demonstrated to have a vasodilator effect. It increases venous capacitance. Left ventricular diastolic pressure drops at a time much sooner than significant net sodium excretion has occurred (4).

The starting dose of furosemide should be increased in patients known to have renal failure. It is unreasonable to expect a patient with a creatinine of 4 mg/dl to respond to the usual starting dose of furosemide. The patient is ill-served by the delay involved in slowly escalating the dose. A starting dose of 120 mg IV seems more appropriate. A summary of therapeutic suggestions is given in Table 4-2.

Once pulmonary edema has resolved, the desired rate of diuresis is slower and the dosage of furosemide should be decreased. Further diagnostic and treatment efforts will depend upon the event which precipitated the episode of pulmonary edema.

Complications of Diuretic Treatment in Congestive Heart Failure

Complications of chronic diuretic use include hypokalemia, metabolic alkalosis, and prerenal azotemia. Metabolic alkalosis typically responds to discontinuation of the diuretic or reduction of its dose for a few days. Hypokalemia is treated with potassium chloride supplementation. With diuresis, potassium loss is quite variable. In the outpatient with mild congestive heart failure, it is usually best not to begin potassium supplements until hypokalemia actually develops. In the patient receiving larger doses of diuretics or in a patient who is digitalized, potassium may be begun at a dose of 40 mEq daily. While the patient is still losing weight, potassium losses can be quite large, and frequent monitoring of potassium will be required in this period. Once the patient has reached a steady state, a stable dose of potassium may be determined and the frequency of monitoring may be reduced. The potassium-sparing diuretics, spironolactone, triamterene, and amiloride may be given along with kaliuretic diuretics as an alternative to potassium supplementation. Combination drugs are available for this purpose. Although they may simplify the patient medication regimen, a valuable goal in patients who have had difficulty complying with their prescribed medications, these combinations are expensive and seldom match exactly the individual doses required for a given patient. Thus, their use is rarely appropriate. The use of supplemental potassium along with the antikaliuretic agents is to be avoided as severe, protracted hyperkalemia can result. Salt substitutes and some low salt foods contain potassium. Patients receiving antikaliuretic agents should be cautioned against the use of these food products.

Prerenal azotemia results from renal underperfusion. It may complicate severe congestive heart failure or be caused by overrapid diuresis with intravascular volume depletion. Characteristically, in prerenal azotemia, the BUN is increased more than the creatinine. This is due to the difference in renal handling of urea and creatinine. Whereas creatinine is filtered and secreted but not reabsorbed, urea is filtered and reabsorbed. Normally, urea clearance averages only 60% of GFR and parallels fluid excretion. In states characterized by low urine flow and high sodium avidity, fractional urea clearance drops even further. The result is retention of urea and a rise in the serum BUN:creatinine ratio above the usual 10:1. With mild prerenal azotemia, only the retention of urea occurs. With more severe heart failure or more severe volume depletion, renal vasoconstriction is sufficient to cause a fall in GFR and serum creatinine concentration rises too.

In the patient with initially normal renal function in whom prerenal azotemia develops during the treatment of congestive heart failure, this complication is managed by stopping diuretics and gently repleting intravascular volume with saline or increased dietary sodium. Treatment is more difficult in patients who present with prerenal azotemia already established. Diuretics will have to be used to treat the congestive heart failure. They may make the prerenal azotemia better if myocardial perfusion is improved or worse if they further lessen renal perfusion. The physician may have to settle for some azotemia in these patients who invariably have severe congestive heart failure. Usually, with time, prerenal azotemia abates and diuretic treatment may be cautiously resumed.

References

1. Cannon, P.J. The kidney in heart failure. N. Engl. J. Med. 296:26–32, 1977.
2. Agus, Z.S., and Goldberg, M. Renal function in congestive heart failure, In: Clinical Cardiovascular Physiology, 1976 (editor: H.J. Levine), New York, Grune and Stratton, pp. 403–444.

3. Puschett, J.B. Physiologic basis for the use of new and older diuretics in congestive heart failure. Cardiovascular Med. 2:119–134, 1977.
4. Dikshit, K., Vyden, J.K., Forrester, J.S, Chatterjee, K., Prakash, R., and Swan, H.J.C. Renal and extrarenal hemodynamic effects of furosemide in congestive heart failure after acute myocardial infarction. N. Engl. J. Med. 288:1087–1090, 1973.

chapter

5

The Contribution of Diuretics to the Management of Hypertension

Beth Piraino, M.D.

One of the major uses of diuretics is in the treatment of hypertension. Before initiating treatment which will be long term, the diagnosis and degree of hypertension must be firmly established. All patients need a basic initial evaluation. Certain patients need a more thorough investigation. In determining whether to choose a diuretic, another antihypertensive agent, or to use only sodium restriction, one must base the decision not only on the degree of blood pressure elevation, but also consider the risk to the patient from the drugs to be administered.

Establishing a Diagnosis of Hypertension

The level of blood pressure called hypertensive is determined by the increased risk to the patient related to an elevation in blood pressure, rather than by the norm of the population. The Framingham study showed that the cardiovascular risk from hypertension increases steadily with an increase in both systolic and diastolic blood pressure (1). For purposes of treatment and definition, certain numbers are useful. According to Kaplan, a male less than 45 yr of age with a blood pressure greater than 140/90 is hypertensive (2). In a male greater than 45 yr of age, the diastolic blood pressure must be greater than 95 to be considered hypertensive. In a woman at any age, a blood pressure greater than 150/95 is considered to be hypertensive. These differences are based on the lower cardiovascular risk of women. Isolated systolic hypertension is defined as a systolic pressure greater than 160 with a diastolic blood pressure of less than 90, and is commonly seen in the elderly. The term labile hypertension is not useful. Blood pressure normally fluctuates since it depends on a number of

TABLE 5-1. Hypertension Categories

Mild: diastolic 90 to 104 mm Hg
Moderate: diastolic 105 to 115 mm Hg
Severe: diastolic > 115 mm Hg
Malignant: papilledema, diastolic usually > 130 mm Hg
Pure systolic: systolic > 160, diastolic < 90

different factors, including activity and emotional state. It may vary as much as 40 mm Hg in an individual during the day (2).

At each visit to the physician, two to three blood pressure readings should be taken and the values averaged. Readings should be taken in both arms since atherosclerotic disease with arterial obstruction may lead to a significant difference between the two arms. In addition, to rule out coarctation of the aorta, the blood pressure in the lower extremities should be determined (with a large sphygmomanometer cuff) at least once. It is appropriate to determine the blood pressure both in the supine position and after two minutes erect. Because of the lability of blood pressure, a patient should not be considered hypertensive until elevated levels have been obtained on at least three visits. An exception is the patient whose diastolic blood pressure is greater than 115 mm Hg, who should be started on therapy at once unless there is some reason to suspect that that patient's blood pressure elevation is related to marked emotional stress. The cuff size of the sphygmomanometer is an important consideration. Too small a cuff may lead to artifactually elevated readings. The width of the cuff should extend two-thirds of the distance between the axilla and antecubital space. In addition, the bladder of the cuff should enclose at least 80% of the arm's circumference and be located over the brachial artery.

Hypertension is divided into mild, moderate and severe, as shown by Table 5-1. Mild hypertension is defined as a diastolic blood pressure of 90–104. Moderate hypertension refers to a diastolic blood pressure between 105 and 115. In severe hypertension the diastolic is greater than 115. Malignant hypertension consists of papilledema associated with severe hypertension. Usually the diastolic blood pressure is very high, greater than 130 mm Hg. Malignant hypertension may or may not be associated with hypertensive encephalopathy.

The high prevalence of hypertension in the United States was shown by a home screening program of 159,000 persons. In the study, 25% of the population had a diastolic blood pressure greater than 90, based on a single reading (Table 5-2). The majority of these patients had mild hypertension. Only 4.7% of the population had a diastolic blood pressure greater than or equal to 105 (3).

TABLE 5-2. Prevalence of Hypertension in the United States[a]

Diastolic BP	Percent of population
$\geqq$ 90	25.3%
$\geqq$100	8.4%
$\geqq$105	4.7%
$\geqq$115	1.4%

[a]Data are taken from reference 3.

Evaluation of Hypertension

The routine work-up of the patient diagnosed as hypertensive should include a detailed history. The patient should be questioned about other cardiovascular risk factors, especially cigarette smoking. Questions directed at determining when the patient's blood pressure was last measured will help document whether one is dealing with hypertension of recent onset or whether it has been present for some time. A good dietary history, with attention to sodium intake, is important. A family history of hypertension, renal or cardiovascular disease should be noted. The patient should be asked whether he or she has angina or claudication. Inquiries should be made about sexual function, since a number of antihypertensive drugs may exacerbate or produce impotence.

Physical findings which are of importance in the hypertensive patient include the presence of bruits over the renal and carotid arteries, evidence of left ventricular hypertrophy (a S_4 and prominent point of maximal impulse), congestive heart failure, and an evaluation of intravascular volume status. A careful funduscopic examination of the retina, looking for hypertensive and arteriosclerotic changes, should also be recorded. Evidence of hypertensive end-organ damage will influence the decision as to whether or not the patient should be treated, and if so, how aggressively.

Basic laboratory evaluation includes a hematocrit, serum electrolytes, urea, creatinine, glucose, uric acid, urinalysis, electrocardiogram and a chest x-ray. Since over 90% of hypertensives have essential hypertension, a more extensive work-up is indicated only if the history, physical examination, or initial laboratory testing suggest a secondary cause (Table 5-3). The majority of patients with secondary hypertension have either chronic renal failure or renovascular disease, such as that related to renal artery stenosis. Evaluation for suspected renal vascular disease should depend on whether or not the patient is a candidate for surgery or for angioplasty and on how easily the blood pressure is controlled by medical therapy. A rapid sequence intravenous pyelogram is the usual first step in establishing this

TABLE 5-3. Etiology of Hypertension[a]

Disease category		Proportion of patients
Essential hypertension:		90–95%
Chronic renal failure:	2–5%	3–8%
Renovascular disease:	1–3%	
Coarctation of aorta:	.1–.2%	.5–1%
Primary aldosteronism:	.1–.4%	
Cushing's syndrome:	.1–.2%	
Pheochromocytoma:	.2%	
Oral contraceptive-induced:		.2–4%

[a]Data from reference 2.

diagnosis, but should not be undertaken if significant renal impairment exists. Other causes of secondary hypertension, which include coarctation of the aorta, primary hyperaldosteronism, Cushing's syndrome and pheochromocytoma, account for one percent or less of all hypertensive disease. Oral contraceptive medication and sympathomimetics also contribute a small percentage of hypertensive patients. Thus, only selected patients warrant an extensive investigation.

The diagnosis of primary hyperaldosteronism should be considered when hypokalemia is present in a patient who is not on a diuretic. Coarctation of the aorta should be suspected when blood pressure in the lower extremities is lower than that in the arms. Normally, it is higher. In addition, the femoral pulses either are difficult to palpate or are absent. Cushing's syndrome may be suspected by the usual stigmata on physical examination: truncal obesity, moon facies, pigmented striae, and buffalo hump. These patients also often have a mild hypokalemic metabolic alkalosis. Pheochromocytoma should be considered in a patient who has greatly fluctuating blood pressures, orthostatic hypotension, and/or tachycardia, and when there is a history of attacks of sweating and flushing. In these patients, a 24-hr urine for catecholamines should be done.

Even without clues to a secondary cause of hypertension in the history, physical examination or initial laboratory tests, a more extensive work-up is appropriate in the young hypertensive, that is, the patient whose onset of hypertension occurs prior to 25 yr of age. In addition, accelerated hypertension or the abrupt onset of severe hypertension in a previously normotensive individual suggests a secondary cause. Both noncompliant patients with diastolic blood pressures greater than 110 and compliant patients with a poor response to treatment should be considered for a more extensive evaluation.

Rationale for the Treatment of Hypertension

Results obtained from a large cooperative study by the Veterans Administration indicated that patients with diastolic blood pressures greater than 115 mm Hg who were treated with a placebo had a high mortality and morbidity compared to those treated with blood pressure lowering agents (4). Patients with renal failure or retinal hemorrhages were excluded from this study. This investigation also demonstrated that the risk of hypertension-associated complications were less in patients with diastolic blood pressure in excess of 104 (but < 115) mm Hg (5). Thus, the benefits of blood pressure control in patients with moderate or severe hypertension are established. There is greater controversy with respect to the treatment of patients with mild blood pressure elevations, that is, with diastolic blood pressures from 90 to 104 mm Hg. Despite the expenditure of large sums of money and a great deal of time, no unanimity of opinion has been reached (6–8). The author and her colleagues have arrived at a treatment program which indicates therapy for all patients with diastolic blood pressure readings greater than 104 mm Hg after multiple readings. If the blood pressure is greater than 140/90 but less than 160/105, other cardiovascular

TABLE 5-4. Guide to the Treatment of Mild Hypertension (Diastolic BP 90–104)

Variables	Consider treatment with sodium restriction alone	Consider treatment with thiazide diuretic
1. Patient age		
elderly	X	
young		X
2. Cardiovascular risk factors		
absent	X	
present		X
3. Hypertensive end organ damage		
absent	X	
present		X
4. Renal function		
normal	X	
decreased		X
5. Diastolic blood pressure		
below 100	X	
above 100		X
6. Relative contraindication(s) to thiazide diuretics		
present	X	
absent		X

risk factors need to be considered. The presence of hyperlipidemia, diabetes, a family history of early cardiovascular disease, a smoking history, or the presence of renal impairment, indicate that an aggressive approach to lowering the blood pressure is appropriate (9). Table 5-4 lists some of the variables to be considered when deciding on the most appropriate treatment for mild hypertension.

Conservative Treatment of Hypertension

If the diastolic blood pressure is between 90 and 104, the initial approach should be to limit dietary sodium intake and to encourage weight loss in the obese patient. Moderate sodium restriction with a diet of approximately 86 mEq of sodium per day (2 gm of sodium) should be instituted. This is equivalent to 5 gm of salt per day, and requires a diet to which no salt is added either from the salt shaker or when cooking. The patient should also avoid heavily salted commercially prepared foods. While a more severe sodium restriction may be difficult for the patient to arrange, the 86 mEq diet should certainly be achievable. A decrease in sodium intake will often suffice in mildly hypertensive patients (10–12). In addition, continued sodium restriction in the patient who begins diuretic therapy will lower urinary potassium losses since distal sodium delivery is decreased. This reduces potassium secretion in exchange for sodium in the distal nephron (see also Chapter 1 and Figure 1-2). In addition, if the patient who is taking a diuretic ingests large quantities of sodium, the blood pressure-lowering effect of the diuretic will be nullified (13). If the diastolic blood pressure remains greater than 105 after 6 mo of attempted weight loss and sodium restriction, then it is appropriate to begin drug treatment. However, as mentioned earlier, if other cardiovascular risk factors are present, drug treatment should be considered for the patient with a diastolic blood pressure greater than 90.

Treatment of Hypertension with Drugs

The diuretic drugs have been successfully utilized either alone or in conjunction with other agents in the therapy of hypertension. As indicated in Table 5-5, a step-wise approach is employed. A thiazide diuretic is generally begun first. If this is not sufficient, a second drug, often a beta blocker, is added. The central sympatholytics, clonidine and methyldopa, and the vasodilator, prazosin, all are alternative agents. The diuretic is generally continued to prevent sodium retention that frequently accompanies the use of these drugs. If the blood pressure is still not adequately controlled on two drugs, a third agent, generally a vasodilator such as hydralazine, is added. A combination that is frequently employed is a thiazide diuretic plus a beta blocker plus hydralazine. In the patient with

TABLE 5-5. Step-care Approach to Hypertension Therapy

1. Na restriction +/− weight loss				
2. Thiazide or clonidine or beta blocker[a]				
3. Thiazide	+	beta blocker or clonidine or methyldopa or prazosin		
4. Thiazide	+	beta blocker	+	hydralazine
5. Loop diuretic	+	beta blocker	+	hydralazine
6. Loop diuretic	+	beta blocker	+	minoxidil
		or		
Loop diuretic	+	captopril		

[a]Because of considerations of frequency and severity of side effects and relative cost, the author and her colleagues usually begin therapy with a diuretic (see text).

severe hypertension not responsive to this regimen, minoxidil, a potent vasodilator, can be substituted for hydralazine. Beta-blockade is especially helpful in counteracting the reflex tachycardia often experienced with vasodilating agents. The diuretic is continued to prevent sodium retention which otherwise can be seen with minoxidil.

Captopril, an angiotensin converting enzyme inhibitor, generally is reserved for the patient with renal vascular hypertension or scleroderma. It is used in combination with a diuretic.

The diuretics employed in treatment of hypertension may be divided into three categories: the thiazides and similar agents, loop diuretics, and the "potassium-sparing" drugs (Table 5-6). The thiazides (and their congeners) represent first-line drugs in the treatment of hypertensive

TABLE 5-6. Diuretics Useful in Hypertension

1. Thiazides and related sulfonamide compounds	First-line drugs in treating most hypertensives
2. Loop diuretics	Hypertensive crises Chronic renal failure Resistant hypertension
3. Potassium-sparing diuretics	Used in conjunction with thiazides in patients with hypokalemia. Spironolactone is the agent of choice for primary aldosteronism.

patients, whereas loop diuretics are useful largely in situations of hypertensive crisis and in patients with both hypertension and chronic renal failure. This group of more potent diuretics is also helpful in treating the patient with resistant hypertension unresponsive to a multiple drug regimen. Unlike the thiazides, the loop diuretics may have to be given more than once a day. In the patient with symptomatic hypokalemia, potassium-sparing diuretics can be given in combination with a thiazide. Classification of these agents according to their utility is mentioned in Table 5-6.

1. Thiazide and Related Diuretics in the Treatment of Hypertension

The thiazide diuretics and their congeners (Appendices 1, 4, 5) have been extensively studied in large hypertensive trials as initial therapy, often compared to no therapy or to other drugs (4, 5, 6, 14, 15). Their utility is greatest in the mild to moderate hypertensive categories. Table 5-7 provides the generic and trade names of these agents. These drugs are generally rapidly absorbed from the gastrointestinal tract (except in

TABLE 5-7. Diuretics Currently Available for Use in Hypertensive Patients

Generic names	Brand names	Usual daily oral dose (mg)
Thiazides		
Chlorothiazide	Diuril	250–500
Hydrochlorothiazide	Esidrix, HydroDiuril, Oretic	25–100
Benzthiazide	Aquatag, Exna	25–100
Hydroflumethiazide	Saluron	25–50
Bendroflumethiazide	Naturetin	2.5–10
Methyclothiazide	Enduron	2.5–10
Trichlormethiazide	Metahydrin, Naqua	2–4
Polythiazide	Renese	1–4
Cyclothiazide	Anhydron	1–2
Related sulfonamide compounds		
Chlorthalidone	Hygroton	25–50
Quinethazone	Hydromox	50–200
Metolazone	Zaroxolyn, Diulo	2.5–20
Loop diuretics		
Furosemide	Lasix	40–120
Ethacrynic acid	Edecrin	50–400
Bumetanide	Bumex	.5–2
Potassium-sparing agents		
Spironolactone	Aldactone	25–100
Triamterene	Dyrenium	100–300
Amiloride	Midamor	5–10

patients with gut wall edema; see also Chapter 1). They are secreted into the tubular lumen where they inhibit sodium transport in the early portion of the distal convoluted tubule (see Figure 1-2 and Appendix 2) (16). The mechanism by which this group of agents lowers blood pressure is incompletely understood. However, it is clear that their effects on blood pressure are only partially related to their ability to reduce the extracellular (and hence, intravascular) fluid volume. This volume contraction is, in turn, related to the natriuresis produced. The thiazides may also cause mild vasodilation, perhaps from an inhibition of sodium transport across blood vessel walls. These drugs also have been shown to lower an abnormal responsiveness to norepinephrine seen in some hypertensives (17). The thiazides generally lower both systolic and diastolic blood pressure by about 6 to 15 mm Hg (18–20). A number of hypertensives with diastolic pressures less than 110 mm Hg can be treated with thiazide-type drugs alone. Patients with volume contraction prior to starting the diuretic generally respond less well than volume expanded patients. Tachyphylaxis has not been encountered. A response is often seen at the lowest dosage employed: 50 mg per day for hydrochlorothiazide, 250 mg per day for chlorothiazide, 25 mg per day for chlorthalidone and 5 mg per day for metolazone. Increasing the dose of hydrochlorothiazide to 100 mg daily may result in a further fall in blood pressure, whereas increasing the dose of chlorthalidone results in little additional effect (2, 21). With the exception of chlorothiazide, these agents have a duration of action of at least 18 hr, so that they can be effectively administered on a once-a-day basis (22). Their usefulness is compromised substantially by renal failure, and they become ineffective at levels of glomerular filtration rate below about 30 ml/minute, or when the serum creatinine exceeds approximately 2.5 mg%. Metolazone, however, may still be effective in patients with advanced renal failure.

Whereas the thiazides have been utilized for some time as initial therapy in hypertension, alternatives to this practice have recently been suggested. Studies have been performed in which the effects of clonidine or beta-blockers as first-line therapy have been compared to those of the thiazide group. For example, beta blockers have been shown to be as effective as hydrochlorothiazide (23, 24). Clonidine alone also has been determined to be effective in lowering blood pressure (25, 26). Therefore, the decision as to whether to begin the thiazides or some other agent in patients with a diastolic blood pressure less than 110 mm Hg must be based on considerations of frequency and severity of side effects of the various agents and their relative costs. Based on these factors, the author and her colleagues have usually decided in favor of beginning with a diuretic (see Table 5-5).

The complications of diuretic therapy are covered fully in Chapter 11, and are usually mild. Lowering of the serum potassium level is common but it only occasionally falls below the normal level (13). Mild metabolic alkalosis may occur but ordinarily does not require treatment. Uric acid levels may rise slightly but symptomatic gouty arthritis is rare. Sulfonamide derivative drugs (such as the thiazides) may cause glucose intolerance which is usually not of clinical significance. Azotemia may develop or worsen (usually because of volume contraction) and an occasional patient has been reported to develop hypercalcemia which remits when the drug is stopped. Rarely, the thiazides have been incriminated in the development of an acute interstitial nephritis manifested by rapidly increasing azotemia, eosinophiluria and oliguria.

The use of an alternative agent, either clonidine or a beta-blocker, is associated with significant side effects. The latter drugs must be avoided or used with great caution in patients with obstructive lung disease, congestive heart failure, peripheral vascular disease, bradycardia and diabetes. The problems related to the use of clonidine have included drowsiness and dry mouth. In addition, postural dizziness has been noted, and is usually seen when the drug dose exceeds .1 mg BID.

In summary, patients with a diastolic blood pressure of less than 105 should be treated with sodium restriction and may or may not require a thiazide-type diuretic, depending upon the presence of other cardiovascular risk factors (see Table 5-4). The patient with a diastolic blood pressure above 104 should be started on low doses of a thiazide diuretic, e.g., hydrochlorothiazide 50 mg/day. If this is ineffective, the dose can be doubled. If blood pressure is then inadequately controlled on the diuretic alone, the next step is to add another agent rather than increasing the diuretic further (see Table 5-5). Combination drugs are available containing a diuretic plus another antihypertensive agent. These have the advantage of simplicity and encourage patient compliance, but they cost more and make adjustments in doses more difficult. It has been our custom to avoid their use.

2. *Loop Diuretics in the Treatment of Hypertension*

The diuretics which impair sodium chloride reabsorption in the ascending limb of the loop of Henle include furosemide, ethacrynic acid, and bumetanide (see Table 5-7). These agents are generally not considered to be first-line drugs in the treatment of hypertension. They are less effective in lowering blood pressure than the thiazides. Their duration of action of 4–8 hr is shorter. Side effects tend to be more severe with greater volume depletion, azotemia and hypokalemia, which are related in part to the ability of these drugs to cause more marked sodium depletion than is the case with the thiazides. Ototoxicity is a real danger when these drugs (especially ethacrynic acid) are given intravenously, but is not common with oral furosemide. Since the incidence of irreversible ototoxicity is greater with ethacrynic acid than with the other agents, it should be reserved for the patient who cannot take furosemide. A newly released drug, bumetanide (Bumex), is now available as an alternative to the latter two agents (27). The blood pressure-lowering effect of loop diuretics results largely from a decrease in intravascular volume.

Loop diuretics are useful in the hypertensive patient who has moderately advanced renal failure and is therefore not responsive to thiazides. About 90% of patients who begin dialysis have hypertension (28). In the majority this is due to sodium and water overload. Prior to the need for dialysis, loop diuretics are often useful in helping to control edema and thus, hypertension. Some patients will not respond to furosemide alone, even in large doses. In these patients, metolazone, 5–20 mg each day, can be added to oral furosemide, 40–120 mg twice a day. This combination effectively blocks sodium reabsorption at multiple sites within the nephron and generally results in a prompt diuresis. Caution must be exercised when large doses of furosemide or the combination of furosemide and metolazone are used, since the resultant natriuresis and diuresis may worsen volume contraction. The consequent reduction in renal blood flow may accentuate azotemia and precipitate a need for dialysis.

Furosemide may also be useful in the patient with resistant hypertension, defined as an elevation of blood pressure unresponsive to three drugs in the compliant patient (see Tables 5-5 and 5-6) (29). Adherence to sodium restriction should be verified by the collection of a 24-hr urine. The patient should be excreting an amount of sodium approximately equal to his prescribed intake. Compliance to medication must also be examined, perhaps by observing the time between prescription refills. If a decision is made to switch from the thiazides to furosemide, bumetanide or ethacrynic acid, the initial dose should be 40 mg, 0.5–1.0 mg or 50 mg, respectively.

The loop diuretics are often helpful in the therapy of hypertensive crises: both accelerated and malignant hypertension (30). A rapid reduction in the extracellular fluid volume of these patients if they are not already volume contracted will frequently result in a reduction in blood pressure. In addition the loop diuretic will potentiate the action of other antihypertensive agents. The intravenous administration of 40–80 mg of furosemide (or comparable doses of bumetanide or ethacrynic acid, see Table 5-7) will rapidly lower blood pressure in a patient with normal renal function. If this therapy is unsuccessful or inadequate, it is our practice to add hydralazine, 25–50 mg orally every six hours or 10–20 mg intramuscularly. Beta-blockade may also be required. In malignant hypertension, the patient should be treated with an intravenously administered loop diuretic plus parenteral hydralazine or nitroprusside (31). In Table 5-8, an outline for the treatment of hypertensive crisis is provided. If renal

TABLE 5-8. Suggestions for the Treatment of Hypertensive Crisis

A. Accelerated hypertension: severe hypertension associated with retinal exudates and hemorrhages

1. Loop diuretic and	for example	furosemide, 40–120 mg p.o. BID[a]
2. β blocker and	for example	propranolol, 40–80 mg p.o. q 6 hr
3. Vasodilator	for example	hydralazine, 25–50 mg p.o. q 4–6 hr or minoxidil, 2.5–10 mg p.o. q 6 hr[b,c]

B. Malignant hypertension: severe hypertension associated with papilledema

1. Initial therapy

a. Loop diuretic and	for example	furosemide, 40–80 mg IV initially,[a] then as needed
b. Vasodilator	for example	hydralazine,[c] 10–40 mg 1M q 2–6 hr or nitroprusside .5–10 μg/kg/minute IV continuously[d]

2. Once BP controlled, convert to oral medications as described in A.

[a]Higher doses of furosemide, up to 300 mg, and the addition of oral metolazone, 5–20 mg, may be needed in patients with renal failure.

[b]Minoxidil can be given once a day when the patient is stable.

[c]β-blocker may be needed to control reflex tachycardia.

[d]Nitroprusside should be used only in an intensive care unit with close blood pressure monitoring. Usually an intraarterial line is required. The dose is titrated minute by minute to the blood pressure desired.

failure has supervened, dialysis may be required. Often, if renal insufficiency is already present, it may worsen as the blood pressure is lowered (32). Care should therefore be taken not to decrease the blood pressure too fast or to levels that are too low. For example, in a patient with a blood pressure of 240/130, one might settle for a gradual reduction to the 160–180/100–110 range, at least in the first several hours. As with other medical emergencies, therapy must be guided by clinical judgment and continued monitoring of clinical cardiovascular and laboratory parameters as well as urinary output.

3. *Potassium-Sparing Diuretics in the Treatment of Hypertension*

The potassium-sparing diuretics include spironolactone, which is a competitive inhibitor of aldosterone, triamterene and amiloride (Table 5-7). These drugs act on the distal nephron to inhibit the exchange of sodium for potassium. They are weak natriuretic drugs and are not especially effective in lowering blood pressure by themselves. They may, however, be beneficial in combination with other diuretics in the patient who has

TABLE 5-9. Approach to Diuretic-induced Hypokalemia

1. Increase potassium in diet, decrease sodium in diet
2. Use potassium-containing salt substitute[a]
3. Potassium chloride supplementation[a]
4. Add potassium-sparing diuretic[a]

[a]Use very cautiously in the elderly and in patients with decreased GFR.

troublesome symptomatic hypokalemia. The serum potassium occasionally may be low enough to cause symptoms of polyuria, muscular weakness and ventricular irritability or other complications, requiring treatment. Even mild hypokalemia should be avoided in the patient on a digitalis preparation. The potassium-sparing diuretics are available in combination with thiazides, or can be given separately. The combinations have the advantage of convenience but are expansive. When using these drugs, one must watch carefully for hyperkalemia, especially in patients who have renal insufficiency or Type IV renal tubular acidosis (hyporeninemic hypoaldosteronism). Less expensive methods for raising the serum potassium include increasing the potassium in the diet, and having the patient use a potassium-containing salt substitute. Potassium chloride supplementation is another alternative (see Table 5-9). Magnesium depletion, which can result from therapy with the thiazide diuretics, may make the patient refractory to potassium supplementation.

Hypertension in the Elderly

A discussion of the management of hypertension in the elderly warrants special consideration because it presents certain problems in diagnosis and treatment which differ from those of other hypertensives. Elevated blood pressure is common in the elderly. It has been estimated that about 50% of patients over 65 years of age have a blood pressure greater than 160/95 (33). Caution must be exercised in evaluating these measurements, however, because cuff readings may not correlate with true intra-arterial pressure. This is the case because elderly patients often have rigid arterial vessels that cannot easily be occluded by the blood pressure cuff, with the result that artifactually high readings are obtained. Such patients can be differentiated on the basis that: 1) their vessels feel rigid to palpation, 2) they respond poorly to antihypertensive medication, 3) severe orthostatic hypotension may result from small doses of medication, and 4) evidence of end-organ damage is not present despite relatively high cuff pressure readings. On the other hand, hypertension in the 65–75 age range is associated with three times the risk of cardiovascular disease compared to that seen in normotensives in the same age group (33). In the Framingham study, systolic hypertension caused an even greater risk in the aged than did diastolic hypertension (1). Despite this observation, controlled studies demonstrating the benefit of reducing isolated systolic hypertension have not yet been performed. Therefore, elderly patients with systolic hypertension should be approached in a conservative manner, including the restriction of sodium intake and the recording of multiple blood pressure measurements before the decision is made to begin drug therapy (34).

Diuretic side effects which include hyperglycemia, hypokalemia and hyperuricemia may be more symptomatic in the elderly patient. The hypokalemia which is often of no concern to the younger patient may predispose the elderly patient to ventricular irritability. Moreover, methyldopa, reserpine and clonidine all have central nervous system side effects which may be more pronounced in the elderly. Also it is especially important to avoid orthostatic hypotension. Beta-adrenergic blocking agents may be used in this age group if no contraindication to their use is present.

If the decision is made to institute drug therapy, thiazides are the best drugs to begin with, employing a dosage about one-half that usually used in younger patients. The dose can then be increased as necessary and as tolerated, but only very gradually, and probably not faster than every 2–4 wk. Potassium supplementation is frequently needed and should be started early, sooner than one would in the younger patient. Systolic blood pressure should not be lowered below 140–160 mm Hg (33).

Summary

In summary, diuretics are important in managing the hypertensive patient. The thiazide drugs are first-line antihypertensive agents and may be sufficient in the patient with a mild to moderate elevation of blood pressure. The loop diuretics, in particular furosemide, are useful in hypertensive emergencies and the patient with both azotemia and hypertension. Spironolactone or one of the other potassium-sparing agents may be added to a thiazide in the patient with symptomatic hypokalemia.

References

1. McGee, D., and Gordon, T. The Framington Study, Section 31 (DHEW publ. no. NIH 76-1083). Government Printing Office, Washington, 1976.
2. Kaplan, N.M. Clinical hypertension, Third Edition, 1982, Baltimore/London, Waverly Press, Inc.
3. Hypertension Detection and Follow-up Program Cooperative Group. The Hypertension Detection and Follow-up Program: A Progress Report, Circulation Res., 40:106, 1977.

4. Veterans Administration Cooperative Study Group on Antihypertensive Agents. Effects of treatment on morbidity in hypertension, JAMA, 202:116–122, 1967.
5. Veterans Administration Cooperative Study Group on Antihypertensive Agents. Effects of treatment on morbidity in hypertension. Circulation, 16:991–1004, 1982.
6. Veterans Administration Cooperative Study Group on Antihypertensive Agents. Effects of treatment on morbidity in hypertension, JAMA 213:1143–1152, 1970.
7. McAlister, N.H. Should we treat "mild" hypertension? JAMA, 249:379–382, 1983.
8. Kaplan, N.M. Mild hypertension: When and how to treat. Arch. Intern. Med., 143:255–259, 1983.
9. Freis, E.D. Should mild hypertension be treated? N. Engl. J. Med., 307:306–310, 1982.
10. MacGregor, G.A. Dietary sodium and potassium intake and blood pressure, Lancet, 750–752, 1983.
11. Morgan, T., Gillies, A., Morgan, G., Adam, W., Wilson, M., and Carney, S. Hypertension treated by salt restriction. Lancet, 227–230, 1978.
12. MacGregor, G.A., Best, F.E., Cam, J.M., Markandu, N.D., Elder, D.M., Sagnella, G.A., and Squires, M. Double-Blind randomised crossover trial of moderate sodium restriction in essential hypertension. Lancet, 351–354, 1982.
13. Ram, C.V.S., Garrett, B.N., and Kaplan, N.M. Moderate sodium restriction and various diuretics in the treatment of hypertension. Arch. Intern. Med. 141:1015–1019, 1981.
14. Helgeland, A. Treatment of mild hypertension: a five year controlled drug trial, Am. J. Med. 69:725–732, 1980.
15. Management Committee. The Australian therapeutic trial in mild hypertension. Lancet, 1:1261–1267, 1980.
16. Seely, J.F., and Dirks, J.H. Site of action of diuretic drugs, Kidney International, 11:1–8, 1977.
17. Weidmann, P., Beretta-Piccoli, C., Meier, A., Keusch, G., Glück, Z., and Ziegler, W.H. Antihypertensive mechanism of diuretic treatment with chlorthalidone. Complementary roles of sympathetic axis and sodium, Kidney International, 23:320–326, 1983.
18. Moser, M., and Lunn, J. Responses to captopril and hydrochlorothiazide in black patients with hypertension. Clin. Pharmacol. Ther., 32:307–312, 1982.
19. Nadeau, J., Ogilvie, R.I., Ruedy, J., and Brossard, J.J. Acebutolol and hydrochlorothiazide in essential hypertension, Clin. Pharmacol. Ther., 28:296–301, 1980.
20. Veterans Administration Cooperative Study Group on Antihypertensive Agents. Comparison of propranolol and hydrochlorothiazide for the initial treatment of hypertension, JAMA, 248:1996–2003, 1982.
21. Russell, J.G., Mayhew, S.R., and Humphries, I.S. Chlorthalidone in mild hypertension—dose response relationship, Eur. J. Clin. Pharmacol., 20:407–411, 1981.
22. Lutterodt, A., Nattel, S., and McLeod, P.J. Duration of antihypertensive effect of a single daily dose of hydrochlorothiazide, Clin. Pharmacol. and Ther., 27:324–327, 1980.

23. Alhenc-Gelas, F., Plouin, P.F., Ducrocq, M.B., Corvol, P., and Menard, Joël. Comparison of the antihypertensive and hormonal effects of a cardioselective beta-blocker, acebutolol, and diuretics in essential hypertension, Am. J. Med., 64:1005–1012, 1978.

24. Morgan, T. Monotherapy in the treatment of hypertension, Chest, 83:419–422, 1983.

25. Thananopavarn, C., Gloub, M.S., Eggena, P., Barrett, J.D., and Sambhi, M. Clonidine, a centrally acting sympathetic inhibitor, as monotherapy for mild to moderate hypertension, Am. J. Cardiol. 49:153–157, 1982.

26. Falkner, B., Onesti, G., Lowenthal, D.T., and Affrime, M.B. Effectiveness of centrally acting drugs and diuretics in adolescent hypertension, Clin. Pharmacol. and Ther., 32:577–583, 1982.

27. Flamenbaum, W., and Friedman, R. Pharmacology, therapeutic efficacy, and adverse effects of bumetanide, a new "loop" diuretic, Pharmacotherapy, 2:213–222, 1982.

28. Acosta, J.H. Hypertension in chronic renal disease, Kidney International, 22:702–712, 1982.

29. Ramsay, L.E., Silas, J.H., and Freestone, S. Diuretic treatment of resistant hypertension, Br. Med. J., 281:1101–1103, 1980.

30. Bennett, C. The syndrome of malignant or accelerated hypertension. Cardiovascular Med., 4:1141–1161, 1979.

31. Palmer, R.F., and Lasseter, K.C. Drug therapy—sodium nitroprusside, N. Engl. J. Med., 292:294–297, 1975.

32. Lawton, W.J. The short-term course of renal function in malignant hypertensives with renal insufficiency, Clin. Neph., 17:227–283, 1982.

33. O'Malley, K., and O'Brien, E. Drug therapy: management of hypertension in the elderly, N. Engl. J. Med., 302:1397–1401, 1980.

34. Rosenfeld, J. Hypertension in the elderly, Kidney International, 23:540–547, 1983.

chapter

6

Therapy of Disorders of Calcium Metabolism and Renal Stones with Diuretic Agents

Jesus H. Dominguez, M.D.

The adult human organism is in a state of zero calcium balance. That is, the amount of calcium that enters the body from dietary sources equals that eliminated in the urine and stool. This state is the result of complex events that occur primarily at three levels: 1) intestinal absorption of calcium, 2) bone remodeling, and 3) the renal filtration and tubular reabsorption of calcium.

1. *Intestinal Absorption of Calcium*

The rate of calcium absorption is maximal in the duodenum and decreases distally throughout the length of the intestinal tract. Yet, the surface area, transit time of digestive bulk and calcium transport rates make the small intestine the most important site for calcium absorption. The fractional absorption of calcium is inversely proportional to the dietary content of calcium and is greatly dependent upon the presence of 1,25-dihydroxy vitamin D_3 (1,25 $(OH)_2$ D_3), a metabolite of vitamin D which is produced in the kidney. The synthesis of 1,25 $(OH)_2$ D_3 is promoted by a detected deficiency of calcium by the organism, by an excess of parathyroid hormone and by a decrease in total body phosphate content.

2. *Bone Remodeling*

In adult bone, this process consists of two cellular functions, bone resorption and bone formation. Bone resorption is carried out by cells of hematogenous origin, the osteoclasts. These cells remove bone matrix and mineral by enzymatic digestion. The calcium released by this process gains access to the circulation and eventually is lost in the urine, unless recycled into new bone.

Bone formation is a cellular function conducted by cells of mesenchymal origin, the osteoblasts. These cells deposit a collagen matrix and new bone mineral. Because both processes are intimately linked, large changes in bone distribution occur without an apparent change in skeletal mass. In adult life, these functions contribute to the maintenance of stable blood calcium concentrations in the absorptive and postabsorptive states and to the shifting of stress zones in trabecular bone. Under extraordinary circumstances these two functions are crucial for fracture healing and the crafting of bone shape.

3. *Renal Handling of Calcium*

The normal concentration of blood calcium is maintained largely by the contribution of calcium from dietary sources, the uptake and release of calcium from bone and tubular reabsorption (recovery) of calcium filtered by the glomerulus. The most important regulatory hormone in calcium metabolism is parathyroid hormone (PTH). PTH is secreted by the parathyroid glands when the concentration of blood calcium decreases. The surge in the circulating level of the hormone provokes the synthesis of 1,25 $(OH)_2$ D_3 by the kidney proximal nephron, increases bone resorption, and enhances the tubular reabsorption of calcium by the thick ascending limb of Henle and the distal convolution. All of these multiple organ functions evoked by PTH restore the concentration of blood calcium to a normal level. The measured concentration of total blood calcium is in the range of 8.5–10 mg per deciliter. Some of this calcium (40–50%) is chelated by blood albumin and to a lesser extent by globulin proteins. This leaves a small fraction bound to other anions and a third fraction (40–50%) that is free, or ionized. The ionized form of calcium interacts with all of the cells in the organism. The ionized form, and that calcium bound to other unmeasured anions constitute "ultrafiltrable calcium." Ultrafiltrable calcium, unlike that bound to albumin, is freely filtrable by the glomerulus, accounting for about 50–60% of total circulating calcium. The kidney reabsorbs up to 98–99% of this large amount of filtered calcium (i.e., for an adult with a blood calcium concentration of 10 mg per deciliter and a GFR of 120 ml per min., approximately 8640 mg of calcium are filtered). Most of the filtered calcium is reabsorbed by the proximal nephron coupled to sodium transport (1). A significant proportion of calcium is reabsorbed by the thick ascending limb of Henle and the distal convolution. A minor fraction of filtered calcium is reabsorbed by the collecting tubule. In the thick ascending limb and the distal convolution, calcium reabsorption is enhanced by PTH (1).

Effects of Diuretics on the Renal Handling of Calcium

1. *Thiazides*

The chronic administration of thiazide diuretics produces a significant reduction in urinary calcium (2, 3). The acute effect of these drugs is somewhat controversial. Experimental evidence in humans has documented both reductions and increases in urinary calcium. In any event, since the acute changes on urinary calcium are small, these findings have very limited clinical significance. In contrast, the sustained reductions in urinary calcium induced by the chronic (a week or greater) administration of thiazides in hypercalciuric and normocalciuric states is an important therapeutic tool in clinical medicine (4). Most thiazide diuretics, including recent additions such as metolazone, have this property.

The thiazide drugs act on the luminal side of the distal convolution. At this locus, they dissociate the reabsorption of sodium and calcium. That is, they increase the tubular reabsorption of calcium and inhibit the tubular reabsorption of sodium (5). The mechanism that mediates this effect of the drugs is unknown. Although thiazides have a small inhibitory effect on sodium and calcium transport by the proximal nephron, this effect is dampened by the reabsorption process distal to this segment. It has been suggested that the hypocalciuric effect of the thiazides requires the presence of PTH. However, recent studies in hypoparathyroid humans has verified their effectiveness in the absence of the hormone (6).

2. *Loop Diuretics*

This group of drugs includes: furosemide, ethacrynic acid and bumetanide. The effect of these agents on calcium metabolism has been studied in humans and in animals. These drugs promote the urinary excretion of calcium. Furosemide and bumetanide inhibit the transport of calcium by the thick ascending limb of Henle. In this segment, the transport of calcium is an active process, independent of the activity of Na^+-K^+ ATPase. The alteration in calcium transport induced by the diuretic is thus not the result of an inhibition of the activity of this enzyme. Like thiazides, these agents also act on the luminal side of the tubular membrane. The calciuric action of the loop diuretics has proven to be an effective pharmacological maneuver in clinical medicine (7, 8).

3. *Miscellaneous Agents*

Amiloride promotes the reabsorption of calcium in the distal convoluted tubule. Its mode of action is probably the consequence of an induced reduction in the luminal potential difference, creating a more favorable electrochemical gradient for calcium reabsorption. Accordingly, the reductions in urinary calcium produced by amiloride are additive to those induced by thiazides, thus reflecting their independent mechanisms of action. Spironolactone produces a modest increase in urinary calcium, the mechanism of which is unknown at this time.

Effects of Diuretics on the Extrarenal Handling of Calcium

Several human studies have examined the effects of thiazides on intestinal calcium absorption. The evidence obtained is both conflicting and incomplete, preventing a consistent conclusion. Animal studies have shown that thiazides do not affect the intestinal absorption of calcium. It has also been proposed that the generation of hypercalcemia seen during thiazide therapy could result from a skeletal effect of the drug. Conclusive proof for this thesis has not been obtained following extensive clinical experience with the drugs. There is no evidence, at this time, for a clinical effect of furosemide or other loop diuretics, on either intestinal calcium absorption or the skeleton.

Diuretic Therapy of Diseases of Calcium Metabolism

1. *Hypercalciuric States*

Thiazide diuretics have been used in the following hypercalciuric conditions:

a. renal stone formation,
b. immobilization,
c. hypoparathyroidism, and
d. osteoporosis.

a. Renal Stone Formation

Of those stone formers with a documentable metabolic abnormality, 60–65% have idiopathic hypercalciuria (9). An additional 6–7% of recurrent stone formers have primary hyperparathyroidism, a disorder in which hypercalciuria is also present. The source of the urinary calcium in idiopathic hypercalciuria has been studied by several groups of investigators. Their results reveal a great heterogeneity in the genesis of the hypercalciuria in stone disease. The accumulated data show that the source could be that of a primary defect in renal tubular reabsorption of calcium ("renal leak"), a primary hyperabsorption of calcium by the intestine, or a combination of both (9, 10). The hyperabsorption of calcium may be due to increased renal synthesis of 1,25 dihydroxy vitamin D_3 caused by phosphate depletion, secondary to a primary renal "phosphate leak." In addition, other investigators have reported an increased excretion of urinary uric acid in association with the hypercalciuria (4). The source of the urinary uric acid is an increased ingestion of dietary purines. It is recommended that the therapy of stone disease be based upon the underlying cause of the hypercalciuria (9). Thus, should the primary problem be an increased intestinal hyperabsorption of calcium, a trial of dietary calcium restriction and high fluid intake should be undertaken. If the problem is that of an increased excretion of calcium from renal origin, thiazide therapy should be instituted. If the problem is that of a "phosphate leak," oral phosphate therapy with or without thiazide therapy is recommended, along with a high fluid intake. An increased urinary excretion of uric acid from a dietary source is best handled by a reduction in dietary purines. However, this is frequently a frustrating endeavor. Therefore, the addition of allopurinol in a low dose is an acceptable alternative. Thiazide therapy is also effective when the primary problem is that of an increased hyperabsorption of calcium by the intestine. It should be used if dietary calcium restriction fails to decrease the increased excretion of urinary calcium. In individuals with hypercalciuria who are in jeopardy for the development of bone disease (such as menopausal females), thiazide therapy is the best therapeutic option regardless of the cause of the idiopathic hypercalciuria. In renal stone disease, the dose is 50–100 mg of hydrochlorothiazide daily. A summary of suggested therapy in hypercalciuric renal stone disease is presented in Table 6-1.

As pointed out earlier, primary hyperparathyroidism is frequently seen in the recurrent stone former. For this reason, every effort should be made to identify those stone formers with that disease. Thiazide therapy is contraindicated in primary hyperparathyroidism because of the likelihood that the hypercalcemia seen in this condition will be aggravated (11).

b. Immobilization

During prolonged immobilization there is an increased mineral release from bone. At least in the early stages, this is produced by osteoclastic bone resorption. The cause of this problem is unknown. As a consequence of these events, there is an increased urinary excretion of calcium and kidney stones frequently develop. Another outcome of this problem is the development of hypercalcemia as well. Recent experimental evidence has demonstrated that a new diphosphonate analog is a very promising drug in the treatment of this condition. However, at the time of this writing, the drug was not available for clinical use. Nevertheless, thiazides provide an effective alternative in the management of hypercalciuria in this situation.

TABLE 6-1. Therapy of Hypercalciuric Renal Stone Disease[a]

Metabolic abnormality	Increased oral fluid intake (>2 liters per day)	Dietary calcium restriction (<400 mg per day)
Primary Intestinal Absorptive Hypercalciuria	First step	First step
Primary Renal Calcium Leak	First step	——
Hypercalciuria with Hypophosphatemia	First step	Second step
Hyperuricosuria of Dietary Origin with Hypercalciuria	First step	Second step
Hypercalciuria in Menopausal or Post-Menopausal Females	First step	——
Normocalciuric Nephrolithiasis[c]	First step	First step

[a]First step is the initial treatment which attempts to selectively address the underlying abnormality. If hypercalciuria and/or stone formation continues despite this action, a second step is then indicated.

[b]Another thiazide derivative could be used at comparable dosage. If hypokalemia develops, a combination of 50 mg of hydrochlorothiazide plus 5 mg of amiloride could be used, or potassium citrate supplementation could be given.

The main problem with this approach is the threat of hypercalcemia, so that close monitoring of serum calcium is necessary.

c. Hypoparathyroidism

Hypercalciuria is a common complication of hypoparathyroidism. In this situation, the use of thiazides in combination with vitamin D has resulted in an increase in serum calcium. Whether the reported increases in total calcium result simply from volume contraction, or are related to an increase in ionized calcium is not totally clear. Both factors may play a role. Two significant problems restrict the use of thiazides in hypoparathyroidism. First, when thiazides are given in conjunction with vitamin D, the risk of hypercalcemia is much greater. Second, the use of thiazides to the point of significant volume contraction is not the best therapeutic alternative for the treatment of this disorder.

d. Osteoporosis

The clinical diagnosis of osteoporosis includes a heterogenous group of disorders of bone. The common denominator for these conditions is a reduction in the total volume of bone. Hypercalciuria has been reported in a form of juvenile osteoporosis exclusively affecting young males. A beneficial role of thiazides in these conditions has not been established in

TABLE 6-1 (*continued*)

Hydrochlorothiazide[b] (50 mg once or twice per day)	Oral neutral phosphate (500 mg three to four times per day)	Dietary purine restriction	Allopurinol 100 mg per day
Second step	——	——	——
First step	——	——	——
Second step	First step	——	——
Second step	——	First step	Second step
First step	——	——	——
First step	Second step	——	——

[c]In this condition, an associated metabolic abnormality is not documented. Frequently, stone disease in this clinical picture is quite severe and resistant to therapy, although the thiazides may be beneficial. Oral phosphate has been used as a non-specific inhibitor of stone formation.

TABLE 6-2. Conditions Frequently Complicated by Hypercalcemia

A. Main source is increased bone resorption
   1. Hyperparathyroidism
   2. Malignancy
   3. Immobilization
   4. Vitamin D[a] or A overdose
   5. Thyrotoxicosis

B. Main source is increased intestinal absorption of calcium
   1. Sarcoidosis
   2. Vitamin D overdose[a]
   3. Milk-alkali syndrome

C. Main source is increased renal tubular reabsorption of calcium
   1. Thiazide therapy
   2. Syndrome of hypercalcemia with hypocalciuria

D. Main source is extraskeletal mobilization of tissue calcium
   1. Postacute renal failure (rhabdomyolysis)

E. Main source is a decreased bone calcium uptake
   1. Mineralization defect in chronic renal failure

[a]Vitamin D enhances both bone resorption and intestinal calcium absorption.

TABLE 6-3. An Outline for the Acute Therapy of Hypercalcemia

Main source of the elevated blood calcium	IV hydration[1] with normal saline solutions	Furosemide[2] IV, 40–80 mg every two hours if needed, to maintain a urine output of 500 ml/hour
A. Increased[5] bone resorption	First Step	First Step
B. Increased intestinal absorption of calcium	First Step	First Step

Notes

1. The normal saline infusion is given first to restore euvolemia and continues, for less than 24 hours, to sustain a urine output of 500 ml per hour.
2. Furosemide is given to maintain a urine output of 500 ml per hour for a period less than 24 hours. These two therapies (1 and 2) must be viewed as supportive and temporary.
3. Could use equivalent doses of another glucocorticoid orally or parenterally.

clinical practice. Some investigators have used thiazides in the treatment of these conditions in association with vitamin D therapy (11). Because of the risk of hypercalcemia in this setting, it is suggested that thiazide therapy be limited to those experienced in the treatment of osteoporosis.

2. *Hypercalcemia*

The causes of hypercalcemia are listed in Table 6-2. The clinical presentation of hypercalcemia ranges from the lack of any symptoms whatever to the patient with severe organ involvement, including acute renal failure, cardiac arrhythmias or coma. The severely hypercalcemic patient, especially if there is cardiac, renal or central nervous system involvement, should be considered a medical emergency, and treatment should be initiated at once. Volume expansion with normal saline is the first therapeutic intervention in most situations, since the patient is most likely volume contracted as a result of both an ongoing diuresis and poor intake. The second goal is to promote a vigorous diuresis by the use of intravenous furosemide (7). This is achieved by repetitive injection of the diuretic at intervals timed to sustain a diuresis greater than 500 ml per hr. This massive loss of fluid with its complement of sodium and potassium must be replaced continuously throughout the treatment period. In patients with renal insufficiency, it is probably best to use both diuretics and saline expansion to avoid cardiac overload and failure. If the use of furosemide is not possible, then bumetanide or ethacrynic acid could be used as alternative agents.

Prednisone,[3] 30–40 mg per day	Salmon[4] calcitonin, 100–200 MRC units every eight hours	Mithramycin IV, 15-25 μg/kg	Dialysis
Second Step	Second Step	Third Step	Fourth Step
Second Step	—	—	—

4. "Calcitonin escape" might be delayed by concurrent glucocorticoid therapy. These two forms of therapy (3 and 4) are given to decrease bone resorption.
5. The therapy for the hypercalcemia of primary hyperparathyroidism and hyperthyroidism should be directed to the primary endocrine disorder.

It is important to emphasize that the diuretic treatment of hypercalcemia is restricted to only a few hours. Along with this therapy, more definitive and longer-lasting therapeutic strategies should be instituted (12, 13) (Table 6-3).

References

1. Sutton, R.A.L. Disorders of renal calcium excretion. Kidney Int. 23:665–673, 1983.
2. Yendt, E.R., and Cohanim, M. Prevention of calcium stones with thiazides. Kidney Int. 13:397–409, 1978.
3. Suki, W.N. Effects of diuretics on calcium metabolism, in: Regulation of Phosphate and Mineral Metabolism, S.G. Massry, J.M. Letteri and E. Ritz (editors), Adv. Exp. Med. Biol. 151:493–500, 1982.
4. Coe, F.L. Treated and untreated recurrent calcium nephrolithiasis in patients with idiopathic hypercalciuria, hyperuricosuria, or no metabolic disorder. Ann. Intern. Med. 87:404–410, 1977.
5. Costanzo, L.S., and Windhager, E.E. Calcium and sodium transport by the distal convoluted tubule of the rat. Am. J. Physiol. 235:F492–F506, 1978.
6. Porter, R.H., Cox, B.G., Heaney, D., Hostetter, T.H., Stinebaugh, B.J., and Suki, W.N. Treatment of hypoparathyroid patients with chlorthalidone. New Engl. J. Med. 298:577–581, 1978.
7. Suki, W.N., Yium, J.J., Von Minden, M., Saller-Hebert, C., Eknoyan, G., and Martinez Maldonado, M. Acute treatment of hypercalcemia with furosemide. New Engl. J. Med. 283:836–840, 1970.

8. Bell, N. Hypercalcemic and hypocalcemic disorders: diagnosis and treatment. Nephron 23:147–151, 1979.
9. Pak, C.Y.C., Peters, P., Hurt, G., Kadesky,M., Fine, M., Reisman, D., Splann, F., Caramela, C., Freeman, A., Britton, F., Sakhaee, K., and Breslav, N.A. Is selective therapy of recurrent nephrolithiasis possible? Am. J. Med. 71:615–622, 1981.
10. Lemann, J. Idiopathic hypercalciuria, in: Nephrolithiasis. Contemporary Issues in Nephrology, Volume 5, 1980 (editors: F.L. Coe, B.M. Brenner and J.H. Stein), New York, Churchill Livingstone, pp. 86–115.
11. Parfitt, A.M. Chlorothiazide-induced hypercalcemia in juvenile osteoporosis and hyperparathyroidism. New Engl. J. Med. 281:55–59, 1969.
12. Canalis, E.M., Mundy, G.R., and Raisz, L.G. Hypercalcemia: diagnosis and therapy. Connecticut Med. 41:16–21, 1977.
13. Rodman, J.S., and Sherwood, L.M. Disorders of mineral metabolism in malignancy, in: Metabolic Bone Disease, Volume II, 1978 (editors: L.V. Avioli and S.M. Krane), New York, Academic Press, pp. 577–631.

chapter

7

Diuretics in Acute Renal Failure

Raymond Rault, M.D.

An abrupt, often reversible, decrease in renal function with progressive rise in blood urea nitrogen and creatinine levels is a common medical emergency. In a recent prospective study, 4.9% of 2,216 patients admitted to hospital developed some degree of renal insufficiency (1). Despite advances in management including the use of early and frequent dialysis, the mortality of acute renal failure is 50–65%. The highest mortality occurs in patients with "surgical" acute renal failure (i.e., following major trauma or cardiovascular surgery) whereas patients with "medical" acute renal failure (i.e., following aminoglycoside therapy or contrast media) have a better prognosis. The severity of the underlying disease often determines the outcome but it would be helpful if the acute renal failure could be prevented or ameliorated. Oliguria, long considered to be one of the cardinal manifestations of acute renal failure, occurs in half to two-thirds of cases (2). Not surprisingly, drugs capable of increasing urine output have been used in an attempt to prevent or reverse this disorder. Two classes of diuretics are widely prescribed: osmotic agents (e.g., mannitol) and "loop" diuretics (e.g., furosemide and ethacrynic acid).

The aim of diuretic therapy varies with the clinical situation and the stage of the disease. Attempts to alter the natural history of acute renal failure can be divided into:

1. Prophylaxis in high-risk patients,
2. Treatment of early acute renal failure,
3. Treatment of established acute renal failure.

Differential Diagnosis of Acute Renal Failure

The term acute renal failure covers a wide variety of disorders affecting the kidney with no implications as to etiology. A time-honored approach to the differential diagnosis of this syndrome is to divide acute renal failure into prerenal, postrenal and intrarenal causes. Prerenal acute renal failure is the physiologic response of the normal kidney to hypoperfusion. Correction of the underlying cause rapidly reverses the renal failure. Postrenal failure is due to obstruction of urinary pathways distal to the kidney and the treatment is usually surgical. Intrarenal failure arises from diseases affecting the renal blood vessels, glomeruli, interstitium or tubules. The most common form of acute renal failure follows ischemic or toxic damage to the kidney and is usually called acute tubular necrosis (ATN).

Rational management of acute renal failure, including the use of diuretics, requires a clear understanding of which of the above disorders one is dealing with (Table 7-1). In the majority of cases, this information is readily obtained from the history and physical examination. A carefully performed urinalysis is often valuable since the urine sediment is usually normal in prerenal and postrenal acute renal failure but loaded with renal tubular epithelial cells and coarsely granular casts in acute tubular necrosis. Red blood cell casts have been described in ATN but their presence almost always indicates acute glomerulonephritis. Renal ultrasonography is both noninvasive and accurate if one is considering a diagnosis of urinary tract obstruction and has largely replaced urography in the initial evaluation of the patient with acute renal failure.

TABLE 7-1. Differential Diagnosis of Acute Renal Failure

	Prerenal	Postrenal	Intrarenal (ATN)
History	Loss of blood, plasma or salt and water. Heart disease. Liver disease.	Voiding symptoms Abnormal vaginal bleeding. Renal stones.	Major surgery, trauma, sepsis. Hypotension. Nephrotoxins (including drugs and hemoglobin and myoglobin).
Physical examination	Decreased skin turgor. Postural hypotension. Cold extremities.	Enlarged bladder, prostate. Gynecological malignancy.	Underlying disease.
Urinalysis	Unremarkable.	Normal or red blood cells present	Granular casts. Epithelial cell casts.
Ultrasound	Normal kidneys	Dilated pelvicalyceal system.	Normal pelvicalyceal system.

TABLE 7-2. Urinary Diagnostic Indices

	Prerenal azotemia	Oliguric ATN
Urine osmolarity, mOsm/kg	>500	<350
Urine sodium, mEq/L	<20	>40
FE_{Na}, %*	<1	>1

$$*\frac{\text{clearance of sodium}}{\text{clearance of creatinine}} = \frac{\dfrac{\text{urinary sodium concentration} \times \text{urine flow rate}}{\text{plasma sodium concentration}}}{\dfrac{\text{urinary creatinine concentration} \times \text{urine flow rate}}{\text{plasma creatinine concentration}}} \times 100$$

Notice that the urine volume term cancels out, so FE_{Na} can be calculated as the ratio of urinary sodium concentration over plasma sodium to urinary creatinine concentration over plasma creatinine.

The most common diagnostic difficulty arises in distinguishing between prerenal acute renal failure and acute tubular necrosis. The chemical composition of the urine has proved helpful in such cases and the commonly used indices are listed in Table 7-2 (3). Unfortunately there is a degree of overlap between the two conditions making precise differentiation difficult and only the subsequent clinical course establishes the diagnosis. There are patients in whom the history and physical examination together with other pertinent laboratory data are in conflict with the results of urinary indices. In those cases the clinical findings are more reliable and the chemical composition of the urine alone cannot be used to make a diagnosis. Prerenal acute renal failure resolves if the renal hypoperfusion can be corrected whereas acute tubular necrosis does not. Some authors also distinguish an early or incipient phase of acute renal failure which does not respond to removal of the precipitating factor but which may respond to pharmacologic intervention including the use of diuretics (4).

Pathophysiology of Acute Tubular Necrosis and the Action of Diuretics

The pathophysiology of ATN has not been fully elucidated (5). Two important alterations in renal function are well established: a reduction in renal blood flow to 25–40% of normal with preferential cortical ischemia, and a decreased glomerular filtration rate. These abnormalities persist for days to weeks even when the precipitating factors have been corrected. Several explanations have been proposed to account for the maintenance of impaired renal function in ATN:

1. Tubular obstruction
2. Back-leak of tubular fluid

3. Persistent intrarenal vasoconstriction
4. Decreased glomerular permeability

Attempts to explain the actions of diuretics in acute renal failure have involved mainly the obstructive and vascular hypotheses which will be discussed briefly.

Obstruction of the tubular lumen by cellular debris and casts is an important mechanism for acute renal failure in some cases of ATN. Animal experiments have confirmed the presence of obstruction by cellular debris, and direct measurement of proximal intratubular pressures have shown a three-fold rise with marked diminution in glomerular filtration (6). However, the paucity of histological changes of tubular damage in many cases of acute renal failure suggests that obstruction alone cannot explain all cases.

The major competing theory is sometimes referred to as vasomotor nephropathy. Persistent vasoconstriction of intrarenal blood vessels, affecting the afferent arterioles in particular, could explain the reduction in glomerular filtration rate. This theory is in accord with the observed redistribution of flow from the outer cortex to the inner cortex and medulla. However, one still needs to explain why vasoconstriction persists despite restoration of renal perfusion or removal of the nephrotoxin. Occlusion of the microcirculation by endothelial cell swelling (7) and tubulo-glomerular feedback with local activation of the renin-angiotensin system (8) have both been invoked as possible mechanisms.

This brief outline of the pathophysiology of acute renal failure suggests some of the potential effects of diuretics. It is, of course, quite possible that diuretics simply decrease salt and water reabsorption without altering renal function. Animal experiments suggest that renal function (i.e., glomerular filtration rate) does improve although this has not been confirmed in man.

Mannitol increases osmolar clearance and raises proximal intratubular pressures which would serve to flush out cell debris and casts from obstructed tubules. The drug causes renal vasodilation and decreases cell swelling thus improving renal blood flow. Furosemide also increases osmolar clearance, but in addition, it blocks the chloride-induced tubulo-glomerular feedback mechanism. This drug also increases cortical blood flow thus improving renal hemodynamics.

Experimental and Clinical Studies in Acute Tubular Necrosis

1. *Mannitol*

In animals, mannitol has been shown to prevent the oliguria that accompanies hemorrhagic shock and to afford at least partial protection against acute renal failure induced by ischemia (9) or nephrotoxins (10). In man, small controlled studies have shown improved postoperative renal function in patients given mannitol before surgery on the biliary tract (11). Pretreatment with mannitol has also been recommended for patients undergoing aortic surgery and cardiopulmonary bypass and for patients receiving nephrotoxic agents such as amphotericin, cisplatinum and contrast media. Few controlled studies have been performed, however, and where such studies were done the results have been conflicting.

Mannitol has been widely used in patients immediately after the onset of oliguria (4, 12, 13). In many instances no attempt was made to distinguish between prerenal acute renal failure and acute tubular necrosis. This distinction was made by Luke et al. (13), who found that 20 of 37 oliguric patients responded to mannitol with an increase in urine output. Responders had been oliguric for less than 50 hr and had ratios of urine to plasma osmolarity of 1.05:1 or greater. Although this report, like most others, was uncontrolled, it does appear that mannitol is capable of reversing oliguria if given shortly after the acute insult. It has not been established whether this is due to volume expansion, simple osmotic diuresis or an improvement in renal function. It is also not clear whether mannitol alters the duration of renal failure, the need for dialysis or the subsequent mortality.

2. *Furosemide and Ethacrynic Acid*

The use of potent loop diuretics in the prevention and treatment of acute renal failure has given rise to much controversy. Pretreatment with furosemide has been shown to exert a protective effect in animal models of ischemic (14) and nephrotoxic (15) acute tubular necrosis. In general, the beneficial effects of furosemide are less impressive than those obtained with mannitol. Moreover, furosemide is not uniformly successful in preventing acute renal failure in animal models, and in some cases the drug was actually detrimental (15). Limited studies in man have shown that prophylactic furosemide (16) or ethacrynic acid (17) can prevent the temporary reduction in glomerular filtration rate that follows cardiac and abdominal surgery.

Numerous uncontrolled studies have described the use of furosemide (2, 18) and ethacrynic acid (19) in patients following the onset of oliguria. The duration of renal failure before starting diuretic therapy varied from hours to days, and the dose and frequency of administration differed widely. Intravenous furosemide was used in preference to ethacrynic acid in all recent studies. The results have been conflicting to say the least. Diuresis occurred in roughly half the patients but the effect on renal function was not impressive. However, one study concluded that diuretics may convert oliguric to nonoliguric acute renal failure, thereby decreasing mortality (2).

Controlled studies using furosemide have mainly involved patients with established acute tubular necrosis. An early retrospective study of 105 patients given 2–3 gm of intravenous furosemide daily showed no difference in mortality between treated patients and controls (20). Patients who received furosemide had a shorter period of oliguria and required less dialysis. However, a later prospective study showed no difference in the duration of renal failure, number of dialyses or mortality between treated patients and controls (21).

Thus, although furosemide produces a diuresis in a proportion of patients with oliguric acute tubular necrosis, it has not been shown to alter the course of the renal disease. A major criticism of the above studies is that the authors failed to distinguish between early and established acute tubular necrosis. As previously mentioned, there are studies (4, 13) which suggest that there is a transition phase between prerenal acute renal failure and established acute tubular necrosis. This phase, variously called early or incipient acute tubular necrosis, offers the best prospects for pharmacologic intervention. It is thus recommended that furosemide be used only within the first 36–48 hr following the onset of renal failure.

Recommendations and Dosage

When considering the use of diuretics in acute renal failure, certain principles should be borne in mind. These drugs may either be used prophylactically in high-risk patients (e.g., before aortic or cardiac surgery) or following the onset of acute renal failure. Diuretics should not be used in the initial management of prerenal or postrenal acute renal failure. In such patients, treatment consists of replacement of deficits of blood, plasma and saline or surgical relief of obstruction. If the above conditions have been corrected and the patient remains oliguric, a trial of diuretic therapy is indicated. At present, there is no evidence that nonoliguric patients should receive diuretics (Table 7-3).

TABLE 7-3. Guidelines for Diuretic Use in Acute Tubular Necrosis (ATN)

1. Prevention of ATN (e.g., aortic or cardiac surgery)
   Mannitol 5% by intravenous infusion
   Maintain urine output of 50 ml/hr
   Maximum dose: 100 gm in 24 hr
2. "Early" oliguric ATN
   a) Patient euvolemic:
      Mannitol 25 gm over 3 min
   If diuresis ensues: mannitol 5% by continuous infusion
   b) Patient volume overloaded or fails to respond to mannitol:
      Furosemide 80–400 mg intravenously
3. Oliguric patient with hypovolemia
   No diuretics
   Replace with blood, plasma or saline

Mannitol is the preferred drug for the prevention of acute renal failure. Dosage and rates of administration vary widely in the literature, some authors preferring to give a bolus, others preferring a continuous infusion. One approach is to infuse 5–10% mannitol at a rate which maintains urine output over 50 cc per minute. The total dose should not exceed 100 gm in 24 hr. Urinary losses of salt, water and potassium must be replaced. In the treatment of the oliguric patient, a bolus of 12.5–25 gm of mannitol is given over three minutes. If a diuresis results, this can be maintained by a constant infusion of 5% mannitol. If the patient fails to respond to 25 gm of mannitol the dose should not be repeated.

Patients who fail to respond to mannitol and patients with evidence of volume excess should receive furosemide. The drug has been used in bolus form or as a continuous infusion, the dose varying from 80 mg to 2 gm daily. Generally, a starting dose of 80 mg is given intravenously and doubled every few hours until a diuresis ensues or a total of 400 mg has been given. The author and his colleagues have avoided the use of very large intravenous doses of diuretics (e.g., 1 gm or more) because of the lack of evidence that these are beneficial and because of the potential for adverse effects as outlined in the following section.

Complications

The use of diuretics in acute renal failure is not without hazard. Two major types of adverse effects may occur: excessive loss of salt and water, and accumulation of the drug to toxic levels.

Therapy with mannitol in such patients requires careful monitoring. If the drug produces a diuresis it is important to replace losses of salt and water to prevent volume depletion. The latter is obviously undesirable in a patient who already has compromised renal function. Osmotic diuresis results in losses of water in excess of sodium so that hypernatremia has also been reported following the use of mannitol. If a diuresis does not ensue, repetitive doses of mannitol will cause the drug to accumulate. Mannitol is confined to the extracellular fluid compartment, 80% being excreted by the kidney in subjects with normal renal function. Retention of mannitol raises the tonicity of the extracellular fluid causing water to move out of cells. Two consequences follow from this shift. Volume expansion, if severe enough, causes acute pulmonary edema, whereas hypertonicity and intracellular dehydration cause cerebral dysfunction. Increased serum osmolality with hyponatremia is characteristic (22).

Furosemide and ethacrynic acid are potent diuretics and their injudicious use may also produce volume depletion unless urinary losses are carefully replaced. In addition, both are ototoxic (23). Rapid intravenous injection can cause transient tinnitus, vertigo and deafness. Deafness is said to be more frequently reversible with furosemide than with ethacrynic acid but both drugs have produced permanent deafness (24, 25). For a more complete discussion of diuretic side effects, the reader is referred to Chapter 11.

Conclusions

Diuretics have been used in acute renal failure for many years although the role of these drugs is still a matter of conjecture. Mannitol and furosemide have been shown to exert a protective effect in animal models of acute tubular necrosis but extrapolation of these results to human disease has been fraught with difficulty. The complexity of acute renal failure in man, the timing of the intervention, and the conflicting results obtained in both controlled and uncontrolled studies have been endless sources of debate and disagreement. Under these circumstances, it would be unwise to be dogmatic, but these drugs appear to have a role in two situations. Prevention of acute renal failure in selected individuals is best attempted with mannitol. Once oliguria has developed, mannitol and furosemide should be used as early as possible if they are to be of benefit. Volume depletion must be corrected before considering diuretic therapy. If the patient's volume status is unclear, a fluid challenge with normal saline may be considered. Finally, there seems to be no advantage in using diuretics in patients with established acute tubular necrosis, i.e., 48 hr or more after the onset of oliguria.

References

1. Hou, S.H., Bushinsky, D.A., Wish, J.B., Cohen, J.J., and Harrington, J.T. Hospital-acquired renal insufficiency: A prospective study. Am. J. Med. 74:243, 1983.
2. Anderson, R.J., Linas, S.L., Berns, A.S., Henrich, W.L., Miller, T.R., Gabow, P.A., and Schrier, R.W. Nonoliguric acute renal failure. N. Engl. J. Med. 296:1134, 1977.
3. Miller, T.R., Anderson, R.J., Linas, S.L., Henrich, W.L., Berns, A.S., Gabow, P.A., and Schrier, R.W. Urinary diagnostic indices in acute renal failure. A prospective study. Ann. Intern. Med. 87:47, 1978.
4. Eliahou, H.E., and Bata, A. The diagnosis of acute renal failure. Nephron 2:287, 1965.
5. Levinsky, N.G. Pathophysiology of acute renal failure. N. Engl. J. Med. 296:1453, 1977.
6. Arendhorst, W., Finn, W.F., and Gottschalk, C.W. Pathogenesis of acute renal failure following temporary renal ischemia in the rat. Circ. Res. 37:558, 1975.
7. Flores, J., Dibona, D.R., Beck, C.H., and Leaf, A. The role of cell swelling in ischemic renal damage. J. Clin. Invest. 51:118, 1972.
8. Thurau, K., and Boylan, J.W. Acute renal success. The unexpected logic of oliguria in acute renal failure. Am. J. Med. 61:308, 1976.

9. Cronin, R.E., De Torrente, A., Miller, P.D., Bulger, R.E., Burke, T.J., and Schrier, R.W. Pathogenic mechanisms in early norepinephrine-induced acute renal failure: functional and histological correlates of protection. Kidney Int. 14:115, 1978.
10. Zager, R.A. Glomerular filtration rate and brush border debris excretion after mercuric chloride and ischemic acute renal failure: mannitol versus furosemide diuresis. Nephron 33:196, 1983.
11. Dawson, J.L. Post-operative renal function in obstructive jaundice: effect of a mannitol diuresis. Br. Med. J. 1:82, 1965.
12. Barry, K.G., Malloy, J.P. Oliguric renal failure. Evaluation and therapy by the intravenous infusion of mannitol. JAMA 179:510, 1962.
13. Luke, R.G., Briggs, J.D., Allison, M.E.M., and Kennedy, A.C. Factors determining response to mannitol in acute renal failure. Am. J. Med. Sci. 259:168, 1970.
14. De Torrente, A., Miller, P.D., Cronin, R.E., Paulsen, P.E., Erickson, A.L., and Schrier, R.W. Effects of furosemide and acetylcholine in norepinephrine-induced acute renal failure. Am. J. Physiol. 235:F131, 1978.
15. Bailey, R.R., Natale, R., Turnbull, D.I., and Linton, A.L. Protective effect of furosemide in acute tubular necrosis and acute renal failure. Clin. Sci. and Molecular Med. 45:1, 1973.
16. Nuutinen, L.S., Kairaluoma, M., Tuononen, S., and Larmi, T.K.I. The effect of furosemide on renal function in open heart surgery. J. Cardiovas. Surg. 19:471, 1978.
17. Stahl, W.M., and Stone, A.M. Prophylactic diuresis with ethacrynic acid for prevention of postoperative renal failure. Ann. Surg. 172:361, 1970.
18. Minuth, A.N., Terrell, J.B., and Suki, W.N. Acute renal failure: a study of the course and prognosis of 104 patients and of the role of furosemide. Am. J. Med. Sci. 271:317, 1976.
19. Kjellstrand, C.M. Ethacrynic acid in acute tubular necrosis. Nephron 9:337, 1972.
20. Cantarovich, F., Galli, C., Benedetti, L., Chena, C., Castro, L., Correa, C., Perez Loredo, J., Fernandez, J.C., Locatelli, A., and Tizado, J. High dose furosemide in established acute renal failure. Br. Med. J. 4:449, 1973.
21. Kleinknecht, D., Ganeval, D., Gonsalez-Duque, L.A., and Fermanian, J. Furosemide in acute oliguric renal failure. A controlled trial. Nephron 17:51, 1976.
22. Borges, H.F., Hocks, J.F., and Kjellstrand, C.M. Mannitol intoxication in patients with renal failure. Arch. Intern. Med. 142:63, 1982.
23. Cooperman, L.B., and Rubin, I.L. Toxicity of ethacrynic acid and furosemide. Am. Heart J. 85:831, 1973.
24. Pillay, V.K.G., Schwartz, F.D., Aimi, K., and Kark, R.M. Transient and permanent deafness following treatment with ethacrynic acid in renal failure. Lancet 1:77, 1969.
25. Gallagher, K.L., and Jones, J.K. Furosemide-induced ototoxicity. Ann. Intern. Med. 91:744, 1979.

chapter

8

Use of Diuretics in Patients with Chronic Renal Failure

Michael Sorkin, M.D.

Chronic Renal Failure: Definition of Terms

Chronic renal failure (CRF) is the term used to describe changes in renal function that span the gap between normal renal function and end-stage renal disease (ESRD). ESRD is defined as the progression of renal disease to the point at which the patient is unable to survive without "renal replacement therapy," that is, either dialysis or transplantation. Sometimes, when renal failure is not severe, the patient is said to have "chronic renal insufficiency." However, for the purposes of this chapter, the term chronic renal failure is utilized to indicate any decrease from the individual patient's normal renal function, extending to the point of ESRD. In Chapter 1, normal values are given for glomerular filtration rate in males and females. According to these data, decreased levels of renal function would be expected to range from about 70 to 5 ml/min/1.73 m^2. At the lower limit, most nephrologists would begin ESRD therapy. It should also be noted that GFR declines with age (1).

Mild renal insufficiency may be accompanied by no detectable change on renal biopsy, even when electron microscopy is performed. Furthermore, the changes in renal function that occur even when disease is advanced may bear only a rough correlation to the amount of damage to renal anatomy and histology. Since CRF is a continuum from very mild to very severe, physiological changes also will range from rather mild to very extensive.

Changes in physiology can be observed in patients with minimal renal damage only by a suspicious and thoughtful observer. With careful questioning, it may be discovered that the patient has had subtle symptoms for a long time. One of the earliest of these is the development of nocturia, since one of the earliest changes in renal function is loss of the ability to excrete a concentrated urine. As the renal disease progresses to ESRD, the physiologic changes become much more obvious (see Table 8-1).

As renal function deteriorates, the kidney's susceptibility to injury by any nephrotoxic insult seems to increase. The patient with some renal dysfunction is at greater risk for developing further decreased function as a result of exposure to radiographic contrast material. In addition, the inability to produce concentrated urine and control renal blood flow make the patient with CRF more susceptible to further renal injury from volume depletion. Accordingly, it is important to avoid situations that may adversely affect renal function in the patient with CRF.

This chapter summarizes the information which is available about the progression of changes in renal function and applies these observations in the development of a rational approach to the use of diuretics in CRF.

Adaptation to Chronic Renal Failure

Diseases affecting human renal tissue that lead to CRF usually result in lesions of variable severity distributed throughout both kidneys, often in a nonuniform fashion. In other words, at any given stage of the disease, individual nephrons are affected in a patchy distribution and those nephrons that are affected may be damaged to different degrees. The net effect of the amount of injury and the compensatory response to that injury is measured as the residual renal function. An analysis of the glomerular and tubular alterations seen in CRF involves an evaluation of adaptive changes on the part of the remaining, functioning nephrons (2).

1. Glomerular Hyperfiltration

Destruction of renal tissue leads to an increase in blood flow to the surviving nephrons and to an increase in filtration rate of each of the

TABLE 8-1. Physiologic and Clinical Effects of Renal Injury

A. Physiologic Changes
   1. Decreased functioning renal mass
   2. Increased single nephron function
   3. Increased single nephron sodium and potassium excretion, with preservation of normal sodium and potassium balance
   4. Competition for transport of secreted solutes from blood to urine
B. Clinical Changes
   1. Decreased renal concentrating ability
   2. Decreased ability to adjust to acute changes in sodium or potassium intake
   3. Increased susceptibility to renal injury
   4. Decreased diuretic responsiveness; more potent diuretics required in larger doses

individual surviving nephrons. This increase in single nephron glomerular filtration rate (SNGFR) also results in an increase in the filtered load of sodium per nephron (3). Even though the total amount of sodium filtered per kidney may decrease, the amount filtered by each nephron increases. This means that an increased load of sodium is delivered to each individual tubule.

2. *Tubular Adaptation*

In order to maintain sodium and water balance, the surviving tubules must excrete the same amount of salt and water that was formerly handled by the entire complement of normal nephrons. This means that each surviving nephron must handle a larger percentage of the total load. The net result is that each nephron rejects both a larger fraction and a greater absolute amount of sodium and water than is the case in a normal kidney. In other words, nephrons in an injured kidney have already initiated a functional diuresis (4). The mechanism by which this happens is not well understood. Each functioning nephron, however, has a higher tubular flow rate and excretes a larger amount of sodium than it did prior to the onset of CRF. Not only does the filtered load of solute increase per nephron, but the amount of solute that is competing for transport from peritubular capillaries into the tubular lumen increases. This may have important effects in limiting the amount of diuretic that reaches the tubular lumen.

As an example, furosemide is highly protein bound. It depends on tubular secretion for its diuretic action since its act on the luminal cell membrane of the thick ascending limb of the loop of Henle. As renal failure advances and the load of metabolic waste products rises, the competition for secretion into the tubular lumen (especially that provided by organic acid secretion) diminishes the likelihood that furosemide will reach the tubular fluid. One way to potentially overcome this competitive process is to increase the concentration of furosemide in the blood. This is probably a major reason that some patients in renal failure require very high doses of furosemide to initiate a natriuresis. Since it appears that a certain number of active chloride transporting sites must be affected by the drug, furosemide must be given to achieve a threshold level before its activity can become manifest.

An additional interesting phenomenon occurs when the BUN and other solute concentrations increase in the plasma. The increased filtration rate per nephron results in a higher than usual delivery of total solutes to functioning tubules. These solutes are delivered in high enough concentrations to account for a solute (osmotic) diuresis. Therefore, the urine output may be driven by the number of osmotically active particles filtered. Thus, the urine flow is maintained by virtue of the filtered load of solute, which partially explains the sudden decrease in urine output in patients with renal failure after they have been dialyzed. That is, the large osmotic load is reduced, therefore urine flow falls.

Maladaptive Functional Changes in Renal Failure

The injured kidney has difficulty conserving sodium because of the increased filtered load of solute and tubular flow rate per nephron. Even if the patient's intravascular volume or blood pressure falls somewhat, the filtered load of solute per nephron usually remains greater than normal. This continues to drive urine output even in the face of conditions that would normally decrease it, and results in salt and water conservation. Accordingly, the response to volume depletion is abnormal since the patient has difficulty conserving salt and water. In fact, if sodium intake is severely reduced suddenly, these adaptive mechanisms may result in severe enough sodium depletion to cause dehydration and hypotension. However, mechanisms to prevent this sequence of events are still present. Patients with renal failure can reduce urine sodium concentration and can decrease sodium output if their sodium intake is decreased gradually. The process whereby sodium conservation occurs takes place only if the sodium intake is gradually reduced over weeks or months.

The Use of Diuretics in Chronic Renal Failure

General Comments

The patient with modest CRF will respond to mild to moderately potent diuretics, as does the patient with normal renal function. However, more potent diuretic agents will be needed as renal failure progresses from mild to severe, and higher than normal plasma concentrations of the drugs will be needed to make them effective. As sodium excretion per nephron increases, agents that provoke only a small increase in sodium excretion will have no noticeable effect. Increased plasma concentrations of compounds that circulate in uremia will compete with diuretics for secretion into the tubular lumen. Therefore, higher plasma concentrations of the diuretic will be required to get enough drug into the tubule so that a clinical effect will occur. In all but mild renal failure, it is best to avoid those agents that interfere with adaptive renal responses, unless there are specific indications for their use. Some evidence suggests that renal blood flow may be decreased by hydrochlorothiazide, and this agent is rarely effective at filtration rates below 20–30 ml/min. Certainly, all of the non-steroidal anti-inflammatory drugs reduce renal blood flow and impair the effectiveness of some diuretics—especially furosemide. Because of the renal functional impairment, hydrogen ion excretion is subnormal and the patient is in positive hydrogen ion balance. Therefore, carbonic anhydrase inhibitors such as acetazolamide should be avoided. It is also worth pointing out that they are unlikely to be effective in this situation in which the filtered load of bicarbonate is depressed. Potassium accumulation does not usually become a problem until renal failure is far advanced (GFR: 5–10 ml/min) unless potassium-sparing diuretics like spironolactone, triamterene or amiloride are used.

The use of some agents must be modified because of certain side effects that become a problem only when large doses are used. The deafness caused by large doses of ethacrynic acid, especially when given intravenously, is the most often quoted example. Furosemide administration has also been reported to be associated with ototoxicity, although with a much lower frequency (see also Chapter 11).

Volume depletion must be scrupulously avoided. Diuretics (and sodium restriction) should only be used when there are definite indications. When they are used, the response must be carefully followed. More than one patient has lost his/her remaining renal function to an hypotensive episode induced by over-zealous sodium restriction or diuretics. Water balance is largely independent of sodium balance and control of total body sodium content is the primary goal. Restriction of water is rarely necessary in patients with CRF, and is indicated only when the patient develops hyponatremia that is not associated with diuretic therapy.

Indications for the Use of Diuretics in CRF

Symptomatic salt and water excess is the most important indication for diuretic therapy. This may range from overt pulmonary edema through dyspnea on exertion to uncomfortable ankle edema. Since edema by itself is rarely a problem (other than cosmetic), its presence alone does not necessitate diuretic therapy. The presence of edema signifies excess total body sodium and water and is, therefore, an extremely important finding. In the absence of symptoms or signs of heart failure, a careful evaluation should be made to determine whether other factors are important in the generation of the edema. Venous or lymphatic obstruction and hypoalbuminemia are important causes that are not likely to be helped substantially by diuretics.

Hypertension, a common reason for starting diuretic therapy (see Chapter 5), is frequently detected before the CRF is found. Therefore, many patients will already be on diuretic therapy for their hypertension before the loss of renal function is noticed. Diuretics are still a reasonable choice for the first step of antihypertensive therapy in patients with CRF, especially if there are clues indicating that the hypertension may be partially volume mediated. However, because of the reduction in GFR, therapy may need to be initiated with loop blockers, which frequently will have to be given more than once daily (see Chapter 5 and Tables 5-5 and 5-6). Important indicators of volume-mediated hypertension include edema and a wide pulse pressure with a relatively mild elevation of diastolic pressure.

Nutritional considerations may be important in selecting diuretic therapy over salt restriction. As CRF progresses, malnutrition (especially that related to poor protein intake) becomes a serious problem. Since appetite and taste deteriorate, it may be reasonable to use diuretics rather than encourage inadequate protein and calorie intake by unrealistically severe sodium restriction.

Specific Recommendations

1) Plans for follow-up should be made before planning the specific diuretic dose and schedule. Items most useful in following diuretic therapy are:

a. Weight (on a reliable scale with the same clothing each time).
b. Blood pressure (recumbent followed by standing for three minutes); observe for orthostatic symptoms, especially when edema-free weight is reached.
c. Edema: estimate central venous pressure by observation of the neck veins; evaluate for presacral as well as pretibial and pedal edema.

2) The choice of a diuretic depends upon the level of renal function. Table 8-2 summarizes the strategy for the use of diuretics in CRF. For mild renal failure, hydrochlorothiazide, metolazone or chlorthalidone may be adequate. Start with hydrochlorothiazide 50 mg every morning (or equivalent). The patient may follow his own weight at home and report at regular intervals depending upon the urgency and severity of the situation. If no response has occurred in several days, the dose may be doubled. If the drug has been effective, the patient should have lost 1–2 kg in 5–7 days.

If there is no response, or if the patient has moderate to severe renal failure (GFR 50–20 ml/min), metolazone in increased dosage (10–20 mg/daily) may still be useful, but loop diuretics will often be necessary. If so, initiate therapy with 40–80 mg of furosemide (or 1–2 mg of bumetanide or 50–100 mg of ethacrynic acid). This is usually a low dose for patients with a GFR near 20 ml/min. The appropriate dose may be found either by adding 40 mg each a.m. until a response occurs, or by doubling the dose to a maximum of 240 mg twice daily. Once an effective dose is found, that dose should be given each time (that is, the effective dose should not be divided). The threshold dose for furosemide tends to become higher as

TABLE 8-2. Clinical Strategy in the Use of Diuretics in Chronic Renal Failure

1. Use sodium restriction only when specifically indicated.
2. Use diuretics carefully:
   a. Avoid the thiazides in patients with GFR values under 30 ml/min (serum creatinine above 2–3 mg%).
   b. Begin with 40–80 mg furosemide depending upon the level of renal function. Increase either by 40 mg each time or by doubling the dose until a response is noted, to a maximum of 240 mg. The effective dose may be given twice daily, if necessary.
   c. Sequential blockade may be attempted with a combination such as 10–20 mg of metolazone (given as a single daily dose) plus a loop diuretic.[a] On rare occasions, 20 mg of metolazone may be required.[a]
3. Avoid "potassium-sparing" diuretics.

[a]See Chapter 2, Table 2-4.

GFR fails. Rarely, doses as high as 400 mg have been utilized with success but are not recommended for routine use. This regimen of progressively increasing doses usually results in a clinical response, especially if sodium intake can be controlled at the same time. A realistic goal of 2 gm of dietary sodium daily is recommended.

If these relatively simple measures fail to produce the desired effect, sequential blocking can be used according to the program outlined in Chapter 2, Table 2-4. It is recommended that hydrochlorothiazide be avoided in moderate to severe CFR, since experimental evidence suggests that it may reduce renal blood flow and since it is unlikely to be effective. The combination of furosemide or other loop blockers and metolazone has been very helpful in the experience of the author and his colleagues. The "potassium-sparing" drugs spironolactone, amiloride and triamterene should generally be avoided in CRF because of the potential for the development of hyperkalemia.

Occasionally, a patient with a GFR between 20 and 5 ml/min cannot be controlled using any of the diuretic regimens and sodium restriction programs described here. Dialysis therapy may be the only method of improving salt and water balance. Acute dialysis may also be very helpful in getting the patient through an acute emergency (e.g., pulmonary edema or congestive heart failure that is difficult to control). Once compensated, the problem often may be controlled using more standard means.

References

1. Rowe, J.W., Andres, R., Tobia, J., Norris, A.H., and Shock, N.W. Age-adjusted standards for creatinine clearance. Ann. Int. Med. 84:567–569, 1976.
2. Bricker, N.S., and Fine, L.G. The renal response to progressive nephron loss, in: The Kidney, Second Edition, 1981 (editors: B.M. Brenner and F.C. Rector, Jr.), Philadephia, W.B. Saunders, pp. 1056–1096.

3. Hostetler, T.H., and Brenner, B.M. Glomerular adaptations to renal injury, in: Contemporary Issues in Nephrology, Volume 7, 1981 (editors: B.M. Brenner and J.H. Stein), New York, Churchill Livingstone, pp. 1–27.
4. Hayslett, J.P. Functional adaptation to reduction in renal mass. Physiol. Rev. 59:137–164, 1979.

chapter

9

Diuretics in the Treatment of Patients with Disorders of Water Balance

Barbara Carpenter, M.D.

When renal function is normal, the serum sodium concentration is regulated very tightly between 138 and 142 mmoles (or mEq)/L. This is dependent upon an intact thirst mechanism (and access to water) as well as a normally functioning hypothalamic-pituitary apparatus which senses and responds appropriately to changes in tonicity, either by elaborating anti-diuretic hormone (ADH), or suppressing its release (1–4). Patients become symptomatic with changes in serum sodium concentration ([Na]) because of associated changes in serum tonicity. The rate at which these changes develop as well as the level of change will determine the degree of symptoms. While tonicity is the major stimulus regulating ADH release, the pituitary also responds to alterations in intravascular volume (5).

Hyponatremia

Diagnosis

The diagnosis of true hyponatremia requires that the serum [Na] be less than 135 mmol/L and that the serum osmolality be less than 280 mOsm/kg. With hyperlipidemia or hyperproteinemia, a false diagnosis of hyponatremia will be made because an increased proportion of the plasma volume will be protein or lipid. The sodium content of the plasma water is normal as is plasma osmolality. With hyperglycemia (or when other osmotically active agents are present in the serum) the serum [Na] will be appropriately low, but plasma osmolality will be normal or high due to the osmotic contribution of glucose.

Etiology

Hyponatremia can be associated with low, normal or high total body sodium and volume. Therefore, the hyponatremic syndromes can be categorized according to volume status (6).

1. Hyponatremia associated with volume depletion

In severe intravascular volume depletion from burns, gastrointestinal loss, renal salt wasting or inadequate intake, the pituitary will release ADH in response to a volume stimulus in preference to maintaining tonicity. This sequence of events requires severe volume depletion involving a loss of total body salt and water exceeding 5–10% of body volume. In elderly patients or those taking diuretics, the ability to retain sodium may be impaired and hyponatremia may develop with lesser degrees of volume depletion. Patients with severe adrenal insufficiency have impaired water excretion as well as urinary sodium losses. These patients may present with severe volume depletion without hyponatremia if fluids have been restricted, or with hyponatremia if free access to water has been allowed.

2. Hyponatremia associated with volume overload

In edematous states such as nephrotic syndrome, congestive heart failure, liver failure, or hypoproteinemic syndromes, the kidney reabsorbs salt and water in a way that suggests intravascular volume depletion. The mechanisms as outlined in Chapter 1 and are related to disruption of glomerulo-tubular balance, decreased renal blood flow with subsequent decreased glomerular filtration rate (GFR), as well as activation of the renin-angiotensin-aldosterone axis. Also, intravascular volume depletion may be severe enough to stimulate ADH release. Patients with chronic renal failure may be unable to excrete a water load because the decreased GFR leads to decreased presentation of fluid to distal diluting segments and inability to generate solute-free water (see Chapter 1).

3. Hyponatremia associated with normal volume

Patients with deficient adrenal or thyroid function have an impaired ability to excrete water and may become hyponatremic with relatively normal total body volumes. Stress, pain, psychoses, and drugs that are used to treat those conditions may lead to hyponatremia by stimulating ADH release. Table 9-1 presents a list of drugs which can be associated with the development of hyponatremia, either by a direct effect to stimulate ADH release, or by potentiating the action of ADH on the renal tubule. Also listed are ADH (vasopressin) and two other peptides with ADH agonist effects.

Psychogenic polydipsia leading to hyponatremia requires a free water intake in excess of the ability of the kidneys to excrete water. Because the capacity of the kidney to excrete free water is so large, this requires heroic

TABLE 9-1. Drugs Associated with Hyponatremia, Classified According to Major Mechanism of Effect

ADH Analogues
Vasopressin, oxytocin, DDAVP
Enhance ADH Release
Narcotics
Barbiturates
Anesthetics: Ether, cyclopropane, nitrous oxide
Tricyclic antidepressants
Vincristine
Cyclophosphamide
Chlorpropamide
Enhance ADH Effect on Hydroosmotic Water Flow at the Renal Tubular Level
Sulfonylureas: chlorpropamide, tolbutamide
Aspirin, acetominophen[a]
Non-steroidal anti-inflammatory drugs
Interference with Sodium Transport at Renal Diluting Sites
Thiazide diuretics
Loop diuretics

[a]Although these agents can be demonstrated to interfere with urinary dilution, they have not actually been reported to cuase hyponatremia in humans.

efforts to drink, usually involving the ingestion of several liters of water per hour.

Inappropriate ADH secretion (SIADH) can be diagnosed in the hyponatremic patient only after the above causes of euvolemic hyponatremia have been ruled out. In addition, the patient must have normal or near normal renal function and must be free of edema. Many of these patients are expanded with water and therefore are excreting large amounts of sodium in the urine (4). Patients with SIADH present with hyponatremia and hypoosmolality of the serum with a urine that is less than maximally dilute. It is important to remember that the urinary osmolality does not have to exceed serum osmolality for this diagnosis to be entertained. The important point about the urinary osmolality is that it is inappropriately high (that is, urine is inappropriately concentrated) for the level of the serum osmolality. Thus, the patient is secreting ADH despite a tonicity stimulus which should cause inhibition of its release (7). This may occur in association with tumors or with pulmonary or central nervous system disease, whether metabolic, traumatic, infectious or infiltrative.

Patients with severe debilitating disease may present with a "reset osmostat." This group of patients will respond to a fluid challenge with appropriate dilution of the urine but have a new set point. That is, ADH secretion will be totally suppressed at a lower serum osmolality than in normals. It is rare for this group of patients to have a serum [Na^+] below 125–130 mmol/L.

Symptoms and Signs

The symptoms associated with hyponatremia may vary from none to severe neurologic disorders (Table 9-2). They reflect the level of the serum [Na] as well as the rapidity of the serum [Na] changes. Early complaints may be vague: headache, anorexia, nausea, vomiting and irritability. The patient may progress to seizures, coma or death. In patients with severe volume depletion, evidence of circulatory collapse may be present.

TABLE 9-2. Clinical Findings Associated with Hyponatremia

Headache
Anorexia
Nausia, vomiting, ileus
Confusion, irritability, agitation
Muscle weakness, cramps
Hypothermia
Depressed or abnormal reflexes
Cheyne-Stokes respiration
Pseudobulbar palsy
Seizures, coma

Evaluation

Evaluation of patients with hyponatremia includes:

1. Physical examination.
   a. Assessment of volume status:
      1. Check for edema.
      2. Look for postural changes in blood pressure and pulse.
      3. Evaluate the appropriateness of the thirst mechanism
   b. Look for stigmata of liver disease, adrenal insufficiency, myxedema.
2. Check for drugs associated with hyponatremia (see Table 9-1).
3. Laboratory evaluation.
   a. Check serum glucose, creatinine, electrolytes, osmolality, hemoglobin, and hematocrit. Exclude severe hyperproteinemia or hyperlipidemia as appropriate.
   b. Obtain liver and thyroid function tests. Investigate pituitary-

adrenal axis (including corticotropin stimulation test) if clinically indicated.

c. Check urine volume, and measure 24 hour sodium excretion (compared to intake) as well as random urine sodium concentration and osmolality with simultaneously determined serum osmolality.

d. In patients who are euvolemic or hypervolemic, assess free water excess. Unless ADH secretion or effect is abnormal, urine osmolality should always be less than 100 mOsm/kg when serum osmolality is less than 280 mOsm/L.

4. Measurements of ADH (not yet generally available) are not helpful in the acute evaluation of hyponatremia. However, they may prove useful in evaluating the patient once the emergency situation has been resolved.

Treatment

The therapy of hyponatremia is guided by the level of symptoms. In an asymptomatic or mildly impaired patient, a conservative approach is indicated with treatment of the underlying disorder and water restriction. The majority of patients fall into this category, in the experience of the author and her colleagues. The patient with coma, seizures, or other severe neurologic disturbances is a medical emergency requiring much more aggressive care. This is the only category of patient that will require the infusion of hypertonic saline. It is here also that diuretic therapy plays an important role.

In patients who are hypovolemic or normovolemic, either isotonic or hypertonic saline is given, depending upon the severity of the symptoms. Once the acute emergency is over, isotonic saline solution often needs to be continued in order to keep up with the natriuresis that will be induced by hypertonic (or isotonic) saline administration and/or to replace deficits. In hypervolemic states (for example, congestive heart failure) or in patients who are likely to tolerate saline loads poorly (patients with cardiovascular disease or with renal insufficiency, the elderly, etc.) saline infusion (either hyper- or isotonic) may need to be combined with diuretic administration. In addition to their utility in preventing sodium overload in this setting, loop diuretics are useful since they interfere with urinary concentrating ability and can therefore decrease water retention even if ADH secretion persists. At high urine output, urine is virtually isotonic with plasma even in the presence of high ADH levels. However, since urea and other non-polar solutes are present in the urine, the isosmolar urine has a much lower electrolyte content than plasma. If the urinary sodium and chloride losses are replaced as normal or hypertonic saline, the net effect is to maintain total body sodium content and intravascular volume constant, but to allow total body water to fall and serum osmolality to rise toward normal (8).

Using this method, a diuresis should be initiated by administering IV furosemide in a dose of approximately 1 mg/kg (higher if renal failure is present). Supplemental doses are given as needed to maintain output above 500 ml/hr. Urinary sodium, chloride and potassium losses are scrupulously monitored and replaced as needed with potassium chloride and hypertonic or normal saline solution. In those instances in which the patient is volume overloaded, sodium losses should not be fully replaced in order to allow the sodium excess to be corrected. Intake and output as well as serum and urine electrolytes are repeatedly checked. The patient must also be frequently examined to be certain that volume expansion or depletion due to over- or under-replacement of salt losses has not complicated therapy.

There is some debate as to the optimal rate of correction. In general, serum sodium levels below 120 mEq/L associated with central nervous system dysfunction should be corrected to the 120–125 mEq/L range over a 6–8 hr period. Further correction to normal can usually be accomplished with water restriction alone over the ensuing 24–48 hr.

Example: A 60 kg man presents with seizures and a serum [Na] of 110 mmol/L. If it is planned to replace the patient with hypertonic saline (3% saline contains 513 mEq/L), and one wishes to improve the serum [Na] to 125 mEq/L, the following calculation could be made:

The mEq of sodium required for correction = 125 mEq/L − 110 mEq/L = 15 mEq/L × volume of distribution. If we assume that the total body water (TBW) is 60% of body weight, then: 15 mEq/L × 60 kg × .6 = 540 mEq of sodium. This would mean that the patient needs to receive slightly more than one liter (1053 cc) of hypertonic saline.

This calculation is only an estimate since urinary losses of fluids and electrolytes will be continuing throughout this period. If a diuretic is given, electrolyte-free water will be lost in large quantity at the same time as solute is given. It is not possible to precisely calculate what alteration of hypertonic saline administration must be made. The key to treatment success is frequent (hourly) measurement of serum electrolytes and frequent examination for signs of fluid overload or depletion.

In the patient with less severe symptoms, therapy is directed toward treating the underlying disorder (as is the case in all patients with hyponatremia of whatever degree) and the restriction of fluid intake. In patients whose primary problem is hormonal deficiency, the replacement of thyroid or glucocorticoid should rapidly correct the hyponatremia. In those patients who have either increased ADH secretion or potentiation of the renal tubular actions of ADH secondary to drugs (Table 9-1), the offending agent should be stopped, if possible. In the clinical setting of congestive heart failure, the nephrotic syndrome or liver disease, the ideal of therapy would be to successfully treat the underlying disorder. This is often difficult or impossible to do, at least in the latter two conditions, so that chronic fluid restriction may be necessary. Furthermore, many of these patients are receiving diuretics, which are often etiologic in the development of hyponatremia (see also Chapter 11). These agents may therefore have to be discontinued, at least temporarily, unless they are absolutely essential.

In those cases of SIADH associated with tumors that are not amenable to surgical cure, removal of tumor mass may ameliorate the symptoms of ADH secretion. Water restriction is the mainstay of therapy in all but the volume-depleted patients. In most cases, restriction of 1000 cc per day is tolerated well while the underlying disease is corrected. In patients who are unable to restrict fluid intake and in whom the underlying problem is not correctable, demeclocycline .6 to 1.2 gm per day will inhibit the renal action of ADH. Lithium has been used with some success, but potential renal toxicity makes it a second-choice drug.

Hypernatremia

Hypernatremia can result from water loss, sodium gain, or from water loss in excess of salt loss, and is a much less common occurrence than is hyponatremia. Most episodes of hypernatremia are initiated by urinary or gastrointestinal water loss which could ordinarily be easily replaced by increasing fluid intake. In those instances in which fluid is unavailable (for instance, to young children and the elderly who cannot make their wants known), or when it cannot be ingested (for example, in the patient with persistent vomiting), hypernatremia may result. If the serum sodium concentration exceeds 150 mmol/L, a search for a possible etiology should be initiated, although symptoms are rare until higher levels of serum [Na] are reached.

Etiology

The causes of hypernatremia can be categorized on the basis of volume (and sodium) status.

1. Volume/Sodium Overload

This situation (which is rare) results from a large sodium load in a hypertonic form. There is usually a clearly identifiable cause which is most often iatrogenic: For example, the infusion of large amounts of sodium bicarbonate at a cardiac arrest; the inadvertent intravenous administration of hypertonic saline during a therapeutic abortion; the use of salt instead of sugar when making baby formula; or the incorrect preparation of dialysate for a hemodialysis patient.

2. *Volume/Sodium Depletion*

These patients have lost water in excess of salt. Fluid can be lost through renal mechanisms (e.g., with a glucose or mannitol diuresis), by severe insensible losses (e.g., sweating and/or water vapor from the lungs), or gastrointestinal losses. Infectious diarrhea, osmotic loads such as lactulose or tube feedings are common offenders in the latter category.

3. *Normal Volume/Sodium*

This group of patients consists of those with pure water loss. Although pure water loss may occur from the skin and respiratory tract, this disorder classically results from a lack of ADH secretion or is due to a renal insensitivity to ADH. In each case, the patient presents with hypernatremia, hyperosmolality and very dilute urine. Inadequate pituitary secretion (central diabetes insipidus) may be traumatic, vascular, infiltrative or infectious but in approximately one half of the cases no recognizable etiology is found (Table 9-3). Nephrogenic diabetes insipidus (renal resistance to ADH) can be associated with several primary renal disease processes, but is often related to the administration of certain drugs or to metabolic causes (Table 9-4). The hallmark of ADH lack is the presence of hypernatremia associated with the excretion of a hypoosmolar urine. In patients with partial defects in ADH secretion, the diagnosis may not be obvious without prolonged fluid restriction, since such patients may present with a hyperosmolar urine which, however, is less than maximally concentrated.

TABLE 9-3. Disease States Associated with Inadequate ADH Secretion (Central Diabetes Insipidus)

Idiopathic/Hereditary
Trauma/Surgery
Vascular Accidents
Tumor/Infiltrative
Cysts
Craniopharyngioma
Eosinophilic Granuloma
Tuberculosis
Sarcoidosis
Pineal Tumors
Infections

TABLE 9-4. Etiologic Considerations in Nephrogenic Diabetes Insipidus

Drugs	Electrolyte Disorders
Lithium	Hypercalcemia
Demeclocycline	Hypokalemia
Propoxyphene	Others
Methoxyflurane	Sarcoidosis
Colchicine	Sjögren's syndrome
Amphotericin B	Hereditary
Chronic Renal Failure	
Myeloma	
Amyloidosis	
Pyelonephritis	
Obstructive uropathy	

Symptoms and Signs

Polyuria and polydipsia are common findings in central and nephrogenic diabetes insipidus. It is only when access to water is blocked that symptoms referable to hypernatremia occur. Central nervous system complaints predominate and range from irritability and lethargy to hyperreflexia, seizure and coma.

Evaluation

A careful history and physical examination as well as a thorough review of medications/intravenous orders will usually establish if the patient has received excess sodium or has gastrointestinal losses. Further evaluation should be directed toward the detection of renal disease, a metabolic factor or a drug that could lead to hypernatremia. The following laboratory studies should be obtained:

1. Blood: glucose, calcium, electrolytes, BUN, creatinine, and osmolality.
2. Urine: osmolality, sodium concentration, and volume.

In the absence of an osmotic diuretic (glucose, mannitol, urea), the excretion of a persistently hypoosmolar urine in the presence of a hyperosmolar serum indicates the absence of ADH secretion or insensitivity to its action at the renal tubular level. To distinguish between these two disorders (central versus nephrogenic diabetes insipidus), a water deprivation test should be performed (4). *This should be done only after the hypernatremia has been corrected.* The patient is given no fluid for 6–24 hr, or until he has lost 3–5% of body weight. Urines are collected hourly and osmolality is determined. When the patient has lost 3–5% of body weight, or successive urine osmolalities are unchanged, a concomitant serum osmolality is obtained and the patient is given 5 units of aqueous vasopressin (Pitressin) subcutaneously, or desmopressin acetate (DDAVP) 40 μg intranasally. Urine and serum osmolality are obtained one-half and one hour after administration. In the case of central diabetes insipidus, a urine which had shown no change in osmolality in response to fluid restriction will show an increase in osmolality after the administration of exogenous ADH. Patients with partial defects of ADH secretion will demonstrate urine osmolality values which plateau at levels less than maximally concentrated in response to fluid deprivation, but will show a further increase in concentration after receiving exogenous ADH. Patients with nephrogenic diabetes insipidus will show no change in urine osmolality after ADH administration.

Treatment of Acute Hypernatremia

Like hyponatremia, aggressive and rapid correction of hypernatremia is indicated if neurologic symptoms predominate. With a slowly developing hypernatremic state, the brain develops so-called idiogenic osmoles as a self-protective mechanism to prevent swelling. In this case, rapid correction of the hypernatremia is contraindicated; normal serum osmolality should be restored over several days.

In the volume-depleted patient with hypernatremia, the first consideration is re-expansion of the extracellular fluid volume. This should be performed with normal saline solution (which is hypotonic to the patient), and only after repletion should .45% saline or 5% dextrose in water be given to restore osmolality.

In the patient with salt (and volume) overload, diuretics should be given to initiate a natriuresis and urine losses replaced with free water. Furosemide or other loop diuretics can be given intravenously or by mouth, depending upon the urgency of restoring normal serum sodium concentration. Urine volumes are replaced with 5% dextrose and water intravenously or by oral water intake. In patients with chronic renal failure and sodium overload, dialysis is usually required.

For patients with pure water loss, replacement should be with solute-free water. Dextrose (5%) in water is given intravenously if necessary, but the oral administration of water is preferred, if tolerated. The free water deficit can be calculated using the formula:

$$\frac{\text{actual serum Na}}{\text{desired serum Na}} \times \text{actual total body water (TBW)} = \text{desired TBW}$$

$$\text{desired TBW} - \text{actual TBW} = \text{free water deficit}$$

example

To correct a 60 kg male with a serum [Na] of 165 to a value of 150 mmol/L

$$\text{actual TBW} = 60 \times .6 = 36 \text{ L}$$

$$\text{desired TBW} = \frac{165}{150} \times 36 = 39.6 \text{ L}$$

$$\text{free water deficit} = 39.6 - 36 = 3.6 \text{ L}$$

To correct a patient with severe neurologic symptoms, 3.6 liters of D5/W would then be given intravenously over several hours. Note that this formula assumes that water loss without solute loss has lead to the hypertonicity. Only infrequently is pure water loss seen. As such, the formula is only a first approximation. Frequent monitoring of the treatment response is essential. In addition, since water losses will probably continue if polyuria or diarrhea persists, these losses should be measured or estimated and replaced in addition to the calculated 3.6 liters.

Prevention

In patients with central diabetes insipidus, DDAVP as an intranasal spray has proven to be an effective method of therapy. It is given intranasally in a dose of 5–20 μg once or twice daily. Alternatively, the patient may be given 0.5–1.0 cc of a suspension of vasopressin tannate in oil intramuscularly daily (or, sometimes, every other day is sufficient). Some agents which potentiate the action of ADH on the kidney (e.g., chlorpropamide) or enhance ADH release (e.g., carbamazepine) have been effective in patients with partial central diabetes insipidus.

Patients with nephrogenic diabetes insipidus in whom no remediable cause is found may present little problem so long as they have free access to water. However, when their ability to obtain water is limited, treatment centers on efforts to induce mild hypovolemia with salt restriction and diuretics. A thiazide diuretic is given beginning with a low dose (hydrochlorothiazide 50 mg, or its equivalent). The rationale for this approach is based on the fact that volume depletion leads to enhanced proximal tubular reabsorption of salt and water. Consequently, less filtrate reaches the loop of Henle (and early distal convoluted tubule) where free water formation occurs. Therefore, lesser amounts of free water are lost.

References

1. Baylis, P.H. Hyponatremia and hypernatremia. Clin. Endocrin. Metab. 9:625–637, 1980.
2. Hays, R.M., and Levine, S.D. Pathophysiology of water metabolism, in: The Kidney, 2nd edition, 1981 (editors: B.M. Brenner and F.C. Rector, Jr.), Philadelphia, W.B. Saunders, pp. 777–840.
3. Lassiter, W.E., and Gottschalk, C.W. Disorders of water balance, in: Diseases of the Kidney, L.E. Earley and C.W. Gottschalk (editors) 3rd Edition, 1979, Boston, Little, Brown and Co., pp. 1475–1506.
4. Moses, A.M., and Notman, D.D. Diabetes insipidus and syndrome of inappropriate antidiuretic hormone secretion. Adv. Internal Medicine, G.H. Stollerman, (editor), 27:73–100, 1982.
5. Schrier, R.W., and Berl, T. Disorders of water metabolism, in: Renal and Electrolyte Disorders, 2nd edition, 1980 (editor: R.W. Schrier), Boston, Little, Brown and Co., pp. 1–64.
6. Goldberg, M. Hyponatremia. Med. Clin. No. Amer. 65:251–269, 1981.
7. Zerbe, R., Stropes, L., and Robertson, G. Vasopressin function in the syndrome of inappropriate antidiuresis. Ann. Rev. Med. 31:315–323, 1980.
8. Hartman, D., Rossier, B., Zohlman, R., and Schrier, R. Rapid correction of hyponatremia in the syndrome of inappropriate secretion of antidiuretic hormone. Ann. Int. Med. 78:870–875, 1973.

chapter

10

Diuretic Therapy in Transplant Patients

Barbara Carpenter, M.D.

The use of diuretics in patients with renal allografts is as varied as in patients with normally functioning kidneys. However, there are some unique problems in the transplant patient, which will be discussed in this chapter. The choice of a diuretic agent will depend upon the level of renal function, calcium metabolism, and the urgency for fluid removal, similar to the factors which are taken into consideration in non-transplanted patients. Thiazide diuretics are seldom effective at a glomerular filtration rate (GFR) of less than 20–30 ml/min. Therefore, furosemide or one of the other "loop blockers" may be necessary. In transplant patients, the serum creatinine does not always accurately reflect the GFR because of depleted body muscle mass. Accordingly, an accurate assessment of renal function will often require a 24-hr urine for creatinine clearance.

Use of Diuretics in the Kidney Donor

Living related donors should be well hydrated to establish maximal urine flow prior to donor nephrectomy in order to maintain good flow in the allograft and to ensure good blood flow to the remaining, and now solitary kidney. The first rule of medicine, however—*primum non nocere* (first, do no harm)—forbids the aggressive use of diuretics to establish high urine output. The living related donor should receive no potentially toxic drugs.

The cadaver donor requires very different pre-transplant management in order to maximize graft function after transplant. A potential cadaver kidney donor should be volume expanded with colloid or saline and, if possible, should be weaned from pressor drugs. The rate of immediate function after transplant is much higher with kidneys from donors who were not on pressor agents at the time of surgical harvest. This may reflect a component of pre-nephrectomy acute tubular necrosis (ATN) in the donor. A diuresis should be established—either with mannitol, which acts as a volume expander as well as an osmotic diuretic, or with furosemide (see also Chapter 1 and Appendix 2). Other presurgical manipulations of the cadaver donor may be done in an attempt to prolong graft function. Irradiation and lethal doses of cyclophosphamide and prednisone have been used to decrease the immunogenicity of the transplant. Although there is theoretic benefit to eradicating the donor leukocytes that may be "passengers" in the kidney, clinical studies have been equivocal. At the time of donor nephrectomy, intravenous or intrarenal arterial mannitol and furosemide are given prior to perfusion with a cold heparinized preservation solution.

Use of Diuretics Intraoperatively

The renal allograft is placed extraperitoneally in the iliac fossa. The vascular anastomoses are done first—the donor renal artery end-to-side with the recipient external iliac or end-to-end with the recipient internal iliac. The vein is sewn end-to-side with an iliac vein. The vascular clamps are released after anastomosis and prior to placing the ureter into the bladder. Mannitol is given at the time blood flow is restored to the kidney. As mentioned above, it has the advantage of being a volume expander as well as an osmotic diuretic. Mannitol has been shown to be effective in preventing ATN in animals if it is given before an ischemic or toxic insult to the kidneys (see Chapter 7). This effect may provide the protective benefit of mannitol used prior to donor nephrectomy or revascularization.

The Use of Diuretics in Acute Rejection

Acute rejection is the transplant recipient's early immunologic response to the transplanted kidney. It may occur as early as the first day post-transplant or as late as several months, but is most often seen in about 7–10 days. An episode resembling acute rejection can be seen at any time in patients who have stopped their medications. It may be a full-blown syndrome with fever, tender swollen graft, and anuria, or it may present with only a rise in the serum creatinine. It is a cell-mediated immune response. Biopsies of the allograft show diffuse lymphocytic infiltrate with edema. Tubular changes consistent with ATN may be present. Renal scan or arteriogram will show decreased renal blood flow. During acute rejection episodes, fluid retention may occur secondary to decreased renal blood flow leading to decreased GFR. High dose steroids, the therapy of acute rejection, will add to the fluid retention. Sodium and fluid restriction may be adequate treatment but diuretics are often necessary. Because of the depressed renal function, thiazides are of little use in acute rejection. Furosemide, in a dose of 40 mg, should be given (by mouth, if possible) and the dosage increased in a stepwise fashion until adequate diuresis is established (see also Chapters 2–4). In patients with marked fluid retention with pulmonary vascular congestion, hypertension, or symptomatic peripheral edema, a higher starting dosage of furosemide or equivalent doses of other loop-blockers should be used. The route of administration (oral vs. intravenous) will depend upon the severity of the complications. In patients with total anuria, dialysis is indicated.

The Hypertensive Transplant Patient

Hypertension is a common occurrence post-transplant, occurring in 60–80% of patients. The hypertension is multifactorial. The recipient's native kidneys or the newly transplanted kidney may be secreting excess renin. The incidence of renal artery stenosis post-transplant is higher when the surgical anastomosis is end-to-end with the internal iliac. However, the absence of demonstrable renal artery stenosis does not rule out the allograft as the source of excessive renin production. Intrarenal perfusion may be impaired from mild chronic rejection (an intravascular ischemic phenomenon) leading to enhanced renin secretion. Acute rejection may lead to hypertension with volume retention. Impaired function from any primary cause (e.g., rejection, recurrent or *de novo* glomerulonephritis) is associated with hypertension. High dose steroids and hypercalcemia have also been implicated as etiologic factors. The new immunosuppressive agent cyclosporin A has been shown experimentally to increase renin production and may be another factor causing hypertension in the posttransplant patient. It is important to point out, however, that hypertensive transplanted patients may have normal renal function.

A search for a remediable cause for the hypertension is often unrewarding. Unless control of the blood pressure is difficult or there is a high degree of suspicion for the presence of renal artery stenosis, medical management is the first step. A bruit over the kidney is often regarded as indicative of renal artery stenosis but is an unreliable finding, since bruits over the graft may be present at the time of transplant. However, a new bruit or a change in an old one should cause suspicion. Medical therapy for hypertension should follow the guidelines outlined in Chapter 5. A beta blocker or a diuretic is the first choice in transplant patients. The choice of diuretic will be guided by the level of renal function.

The Transplant Patient with Edema or Nephrotic Syndrome

Transplant patients may have small amounts of pretibial edema without any obvious cause. This may be due to a mild degree of sodium retention. Interruption of lymphatics at the time of surgery may cause unilateral edema in the leg on the side of the transplant allograft. Modest sodium restriction and elevation of the legs will be all that is required.

Full-blown nephrotic syndrome occurs infrequently post-transplant. The disease which caused the failure of the native kidneys may recur in the transplant. This occurs most commonly with focal sclerosis, but recurrent membrano-proliferative glomerulonephritis and membranous glomerulonephritis have been described. *De novo* glomerulonephritis (that is a primary glomerulopathy) may occur unrelated to the original disease. As more transplant biopsies are performed, this is becoming a more frequently recognized complication. Chronic rejection, an indolent, usually progressive process, has been recognized as a cause of the nephrotic syndrome. The treatment for the glomerulopathy in patients with recurrent or *de novo* disease is unclear, as most cases have developed while the patient is taking steroids which are usually the first-line drug for treatment of glomerular disease. The symptomatic treatment of edema is as described in Chapter 2. Sodium restriction, high protein diet, and diuretics will often ameliorate the symptoms of continued protein loss even if the underlying disease process cannot be treated. Transplant nephrectomy has been suggested in patients with severe protein loss but should be reserved for extreme cases.

Hypercalcemia in Transplant Patients

Hypercalcemia post-transplant occurs in 10–30% of patients. It is usually transient, resolving in 6–12 mo, and requires little evaluation or treatment. Severe hypercalcemia after transplant occurs rarely but has been described in patients receiving long-acting vitamin D metabolites and in patients who have paid little attention to calcium and phosphate management prior to transplantation. In most cases, hypercalcemia and hypophosphatemia reflect increased parathyroid hormone (PTH) secretion from hyperplastic glands with a now responsive new kidney. The PTH secretion will normalize in the majority of patients within several months post-transplant. In those who remain mildly hypercalcemic, a trial of conservative therapy is warranted. Phosphate supplements with adequate fluids may be all that is needed. However, prolonged severe hypercalcemia will require a parathyroidectomy. Thiazide diuretics which may accentuate the hypercalcemia should not be used in these patients. In patients who are initially normocalcemic, serum calcium should be checked periodically if therapy with a thiazide diuretic is started. Hypercalcemia which occurs late in the post-transplant course is unusual and deserves a full work-up as outlined in Chapter 6. It is particularly worrisome in transplant patients who are at a higher than average risk for developing malignancies.

Special Problems Related to Diuretic Administration in Transplant Patients

Rapid changes in renal function may occur in patients with renal allografts. Therefore, diuretics which were effective in the steady state may not be effective during a rejection episode. Conversely, high doses of diuretics, necessary during a period of decreased function, may become suddenly more effective as the renal function improves, leading to severe volume depletion. During periods of fluctuating renal function it is best to make decisions about diuretic use on a daily basis.

Patients with abnormal calcium and phosphate metabolism post-transplant may be more sensitive to the hypercalcemic effects of the thiazide drugs. As discussed above, serum calcium should be monitored carefully when therapy with the thiazide diuretics or their congeners is instituted.

Thiazides may be the cause of an increased uric acid. Asymptomatic hyperuricemia should not be treated. Allopurinol therapy is particularly dangerous in patients receiving azathioprine (AZA) as part of the immunosuppressive regime. AZA is a purine analogue and with inhibition of purine metabolism by allopurinol, toxic levels of AZA are rapidly attained with subsequent bone marrow depression.

References

1. Ingelfinger, J.R., Grupe, W.E., and Levey, R.H. Post transplant hypertension in the absence of rejection or recurrent disease. Clinical Nephrology, 15:5:236–239, 1981.
2. Parfitt, A.M. Hypercalcemic hyperparathyroidism following renal transplantation. Mineral Electrolyte Metab., 8:92:112, 1981.
3. Strom, T.B., Tilney, N.L., and Merrill, J.P. Renal transplantation: Clinical management of the transplant patient, Chapter 51, In: The Kidney, 2nd edition, 1981 (editors: B.M. Brenner and F.C. Rector, Jr.), Philadelphia, W.B. Saunders, pp. 2618–2658.
4. Woo, K.T., Yeung, C.K., D'Apice, A.J.F., and Kincaid-Smith, P. Transplant renal artery stenosis. Aust. N. Z. J. Surg., 49 6:613–616, 1979.

chapter

11

Complications of Diuretic Drugs

Marcia R. Silver, M.D.

Diuretics are among the most frequently prescribed drugs in the United States (1) and, in general, are safe and well tolerated. Their use is nonetheless associated with numerous complications, which will be discussed in this chapter. These potential and fairly common complications make imperative cautious and judicious prescribing practices and close monitoring of patients taking diuretics.

Hemodynamic Complications

Excessively rapid mobilization of edema fluid, or use of diuretics in patients who are not really volume overloaded, may lead to troublesome symptoms. Patients may complain of fatigue, malaise, weakness, and/or postural dizziness or lightheadedness. Most often, these patients can be shown to have a rise in pulse with standing, with or without a fall in blood pressure, indicative of volume depletion. They may be thirsty and may have poor skin turgor, dry mouth, and decreased perspiration. Occasionally, asthenic symptoms may appear in patients who still have edema. Such patients may nonetheless have postural tachycardia and/or hypotension—probably indicating intravascular volume depletion from too rapid diuresis. Discontinuation of diuretics and liberalization of salt and water intake are the appropriate therapeutic steps and usually suffice. Sometimes volume depleted patients have more severe symptoms. They may present with nausea, vomiting, and prostration, and may require IV fluids (usually normal saline) as well as discontinuation of diuretic drugs. These patients usually also have one or more of the metabolic complications described in the sections below, e.g., metabolic alkalosis, hypokalemia. In patients with signs of intravascular volume depletion, one must always consider the possible presence of other causes of volume loss, such as GI bleeding or diarrhea.

Metabolic Complications

1. *Metabolic alkalosis* is probably the most common metabolic complication of diuretic use. It may occur with the use of all of the diuretics that increase excretion of sodium chloride and water, but not bicarbonate, or which induce a substantially greater chloruresis than bicarbonaturia. The only commonly used diuretic which produces different effects on acid-base balance is acetazolamide. The latter drug enhances the excretion of bicarbonate and causes metabolic acidosis rather than alkalosis.

Metabolic alkalosis should be thought of in terms of 1) the circumstances *initiating* or *generating* a primary increase in the plasma bicarbonate concentration and 2) the circumstances causing *maintenance* of the state of metabolic alkalosis. The initiation of a metabolic alkalosis may be caused by 1) loss of hydrogen ion, 2) addition of bicarbonate, or 3) loss of fluid containing disproportionately more chloride than bicarbonate as compared with the extracellular fluid (ECF). Diuretics are often the cause of metabolic alkalosis initiated by these mechanisms because most diuretic-induced volume depletion leads to secondary hyperaldosteronism and renal hydrogen ion loss. In addition, most diuretics cause substantial losses of water containing sodium and chloride but little bicarbonate (2, 3). The losses of sodium chloride and water may occur from multiple sites along the nephron (see Chapter 1), including the proximal tubules, distal tubules, and, perhaps most commonly, the ascending limb of the loop of Henle.

Key to maintenance of the state of metabolic alkalosis is the accompanying volume contraction. The renal response to volume contraction is to avidly reabsorb sodium and water, especially in the proximal tubules. To preserve electroneutrality, every sodium cation reabsorbed must be accompanied by an anion or exchanged for hydrogen (or potassium) ion. This process of hydrogen ion secretion results indirectly in bicarbonate reabsorption. Because the initiating fluid losses included much more chloride than bicarbonate, there is now insufficient chloride available for reabsorption with sodium in the tubules, and therefore significant amounts of sodium are reabsorbed in parallel with hydrogen ion secretion. Thus, bicarbonate reabsorption is stimulated. This is perhaps contrary to what we might expect; the high bicarbonate level ought to lead to renal loss of bicarbonate in order to reestablish a normal pH. But the body seems to place the defense of volume above that of electrolyte or acid-base balance. Therefore, in the volume contracted state, the bulk reabsorption of sodium proximally proceeds avidly and leads to substantial bicarbonate reabsorption because there is insufficient chloride available to accompany the sodium cation. Thus, the acid-base disturbance is perpetuated.

An additional response to volume contraction is increased secretion of aldosterone. This causes increased reabsorption of sodium at distal sites, in exchange for hydrogen and potassium. The resultant increased secretion of potassium may lead to hypokalemia (see below), and the secretion of hydrogen ion leads to further addition of bicarbonate to the extracellular fluid.

The symptoms of metabolic alkalosis are few, and findings are more often related to volume contraction (described above) than to alkalosis. Patients may complain of muscle cramps and weakness. They may have tetany or hyperactive reflexes because alkalemia reduces the ionized fraction of calcium. Severe alkalemia (pH $>$ 7.55) may occasionally be associated with cardiac arrhythmias. Some patients with lung disease may suffer from hypoxemia resulting from the depression of ventilation caused by compensation from metabolic alkalosis.

Treatment of metabolic alkalosis should include discontinuation of diuretics, identification and correction of any other contributing factors (e.g., diarrhea, vomiting, villous adenoma, etc.), and restoration of ample volume and sodium chloride. The chloride is key, for so long as there are insufficient chloride ions available for reabsorption with sodium ions, the kidney will continue to reabsorb bicarbonate and perpetuate the alkalosis. Vigorous volume repletion will also decrease the stimuli for avid proximal reabsorption and aldosterone secretion. Once adequate volume, sodium, and chloride levels are restored, most patients, including those with fairly substantial decreases in GFR, will rapidly excrete the excess extracellular fluid bicarbonate.

2. *Metabolic acidosis* occurs as a complication with only one of the commonly used diuretics, acetazolamide. The acidosis that occurs is really an *expected* result of the action of the drug, which is a carbonic anhydrase inhibitor. It therefore interferes with the normal mechanism for bicarbonate reclamation (largely in the proximal tubules) and causes dumping of bicarbonate by the kidneys. The drug is less effective as a diuretic in the presence of acidosis (since the amount of filtered bicarbonate is reduced), a factor which may in part explain its infrequent use.

3. *Hypokalemia* is a common complication of diuretic use. Most diuretics cause increased excretion of potassium. This is because most diuretics impair sodium chloride transport at a site in the nephron proximal to the sodium-potassium-hydrogen exchange sites in the late distal nephron (see Chapter 1). The presentation of additional sodium ions to these sites leads to increased potassium secretion. If volume contraction has occurred, the increased aldosterone secretion which results will abet this process. Those drugs known as the "potassium-sparing" diuretics, i.e., triamterene,

spironolactone, and amiloride, represent exceptions to the general rule that diuretics generally induce hypokalemia. These drugs are discussed in greater detail below.

Hypokalemia may cause one or more of the following: muscular weakness (sometimes severe enough to cause respiratory depression and/or quadriplegia), orthostatic hypotension, glucose intolerance, ileus, and polyuria. Hypokalemic patients are at increased risk for developing rhabdomyolysis. Many have ECG abnormalities, including flattened T waves, U waves, S-T segment depression, and occasionally arrhythmias. The latter are more common in patients receiving digitalis. Hypokalemia increases renal ammonia production and may thereby worsen hepatic encephalopathy.

Hypokalemia is often associated with metabolic alkalosis. If the patient is volume contracted, the resultant increased aldosterone secretion leads to increased renal potassium losses as described above. Conversely, when patients with high aldosterone levels (e.g., with congestive heart failure, nephrosis, cirrhosis) are given diuretics, they are at increased risk of developing significant hypokalemia.

The safest way to replenish potassium supplies is by mouth. When that is not possible, intravenous potassium may be given safely at a rate of no more than 10 mEq per hr. Rarely, when the complications of severe hypokalemia are acutely life-threatening, up to 40 mEq per hour may be given only with careful monitoring of the ECG and of serum potassium concentrations. When hypokalemia is associated with metabolic alkalosis, it is important to replace the potassium deficit with the *chloride* salt of potassium. Replacement with any alkaline potassium salts (e.g., gluconate, citrate, bicarbonate) will fail to correct the alkalosis and lead to both a perpetuation of the alkalosis and increased potassium losses. The diuretics should be discontinued if the hypokalemia is severe or if the patient is volume depleted.

4. *Hyperkalemia* is seen as a complication of use of the "potassium-sparing" diuretics, spironolactone, triamterene, and amiloride. Although hyperkalemic patients are usually without symptoms, occasional patients complain of weakness, and paralysis rarely may ensue. Lethargy may be an important clue to severe hyperkalemia. More commonly seen are ECG changes which include tall, peaked T waves and decreased R wave amplitude. These are followed, as the potassium rises further, by widening of the QRS complex, prolongation of the P–R interval, and decreased P wave amplitude. Finally, degeneration of the ECG pattern occurs, forming the classic sine wave pattern of hyperkalemia. Cardiac arrest or ventricular arrhythmias may occur in hyperkalemic patients without warning and at *any* point during the progression of ECG changes. Cardiac arrest or life-threatening ventricular arrhythmias are much more common and more

unpredictable in hyperkalemia than in hypokalemia—hence the urgency of treating hyperkalemia and the importance of avoiding it.

Patients with renal impairment, even if not very severe, are at increased risk of developing hyperkalemia with potassium-sparing diuretics. Diabetics also seem to be at increased risk, possibly because many are deficient in renin and aldosterone, as well as having altered insulin responsiveness. Potassium supplementation is rarely appropriate and should be undertaken with great caution in patients taking potassium-sparing diuretics. Salt substitutes are usually potassium chloride, and may cause hyperkalemia when used with potassium-sparing diuretics. Also, the risk of hyperkalemia is increased with volume depletion or any other state which decreases the rate of urine flow or the distal delivery of sodium (all of which decrease potassium excretion).

Hyperkalemia may be treated in several ways. In an urgent situation, calcium gluconate given intravenously will often produce rapid reversal of ECG changes. Glucose and insulin infusions will help move potassium into cells. Bicarbonate infusion (especially in the acidemic patient) is an excellent method of acutely reducing serum potassium by shifting it into cells. These measures are all temporary, lasting up to a few hours. Definitive treatment requires efforts to enhance potassium excretion or to remove potassium from the body by other means. Volume repletion and a thiazide or potent loop diuretic will work well in patients with adequate renal function. Ion exchange resins (e.g., Kayexalate) or dialysis may be required if renal function is inadequate.

5. *Hyponatremia* may be seen in association with diuretic use (4, 5). It may be mild and relatively slow to evolve in association with volume contraction. In this circumstance, the volume stimulus to ADH overrides that of osmolality, leading to conservation of water despite hyponatremia. Hypokalemia appears to enhance this effect, sometimes leading to substantially elevated ADH levels in the presence of only minimal volume deficits. In addition, many diuretics act in the loop and/or distal diluting sites in the nephron, leading to impairments in free water excretion.

Any patient presenting with hyponatremia who has been taking a diuretic, even if only for a few days, should have that drug stopped promptly. The usual assessment of volume status applied to the analysis of hyponatremia should then serve as a guide to treatment (see Chapter 9).

There are other metabolic complications of diuretic use. *Magnesium deficiency* may result from increased magnesium excretion caused by diuretics, usually in the setting of poor intake. Seizures occasionally occur with hypomagnesemia. Hypocalcemia may be refractory to correction with calcium salts in the presence of low magnesium concentrations. Hypomagnesemia probably inhibits parathyroid hormone (PTH) release and bone responsiveness to PTH. Correction of hypomagnesemia usually leads to easy correction of hypocalcemia as well.

Uric acid excretion is inhibited by the thiazides and the potent loop diuretics. Usually the result is only a small increase in serum uric acid concentration without other sequelae, but occasionally acute gout occurs. Gout is an indication for treatment with allopurinol to reduce urate production. Treatment of asymptomatic hyperuricemia in an attempt to prevent gout or chronic urate nephropathy is more controversial. Most nephrologists would not consider treatment of asymptomatic hyperuricemia unless the urate level is persistently above 12 mg/dl. An alternative would be to switch from sulfonamide derivative diuretics to some other class of drugs or to discontinue diuretics entirely (e.g., in hypertension).

The thiazide diuretics decrease *calcium excretion*, an effect which may be used to advantage (see Chapter 6), but which may occasionally lead to hypercalcemia. The potent loop diuretics (e.g., furosemide and bumetanide) increase calcium excretion.

Mild glucose intolerance may be seen with many diuretics that are sulfonamide derivatives. This effect is well described with the thiazides and with furosemide, and may, in part, be due to associated hypokalemia. However, it has not been seen with bumetanide or acetazolamide.

Allergic Complications

Patients who are allergic to sulfonamides are probably at increased risk of allergic reactions to diuretics which are sulfonamide derivatives. These include the thiazides, furosemide, bumetanide, and acetazolamide. Such cross reactions are not common, however, and a cautious clinical trial is appropriate when diuretic use is indicated. Fever, skin rash, bone marrow depression, and allergic interstitial nephritis may be seen in these cases. One or any combination of these manifestations may appear. Thrombocytopenia may be a more common manifestation. Whether the bone marrow effects are truly on an allergic basis is not clearly known. Similarly, the hepatic dysfunction that is occasionally seen with these drugs may be either on an allergic or idiosyncratic basis. Acute interstitial nephritis has been described most commonly in association with the thiazides and with furosemide (6). Definitive diagnosis is made by renal biopsy, and complete recovery may be expected after discontinuation of the offending drug.

Ototoxicity

Ototoxicity associated with diuretic use was first described with ethacrynic acid. Tinnitus and hearing loss were seen, especially when large parenteral doses of the drug were given to patients with renal impairment and/or in association with other nephrotoxic or ototoxic drugs. Although no careful clinical studies have been reported, clinical experience suggests that furosemide is substantially less ototoxic than ethacynic acid, and this observation probably explains the fact that furosemide has essentially replaced ethacrynic acid in clinical use. Curiously, there has been no careful study of furosemide's clinical ototoxicity either. However, it is one of the most commonly prescribed drugs in the United States (1) and the case reports of ototoxicity with furosemide number only about 40. Large parenteral doses and the presence of renal impairment and/or other nephrotoxic or ototoxic drugs are thought to increase the likelihood of ototoxicity. Rapid intravenous infusion may also be a factor. In experiments with dogs, cats, and guinea pigs, the newer potent loop diuretic, bumetanide, appears to be less ototoxic than furosemide when compared on the basis of equivalent diuretic doses. Caution must be exercised in extrapolating these results to man as important interspecies variation has been documented in studies of ototoxicity of other agents. Studies are in progress to attempt to determine whether such a difference can be demonstrated in clinical use.

TABLE 11-1. Some Potential Complications of Diuretics

	Acidosis	Alkalosis	Hyperkalemia	Hypokalemia	Hyperglycemia	Hypercalcemia	Hyperuricemia	Thrombocytopenia	Interstitial nephritis	Ototoxicity	Other
Hydrochlorothiazide[a]		X		X	X	X	X	X	X		Acute pancreatitis
Metolazone[a]		X		X	X		X				
Acetazolamide[a]	X			X				X			Paresthesias, somnolence
Furosemide[a]		X		X	X		X	X	X	X	
Bumetanide[a]		X		X	X		X	X		X	
Ethacrynic acid		X		X			X			X	Severe watery diarrhea
Spironolactone	X		X								Gynecomastia Occasional impotence
Triamterene	X		X				X		X		Weak folic acid antagonist Blood dyscrasias
Amiloride			X								Possibly impotence

[a]Sulfonamide derivative.

Miscellaneous

There are many other unusual adverse effects that have been described in association with use of the various diuretics. Extensive lists are available in standard references (7, 8). A few of these adverse effects are worth mentioning here:

1. paresthesias and somnolence are seen with use of large doses of acetazolamide;
2. acute pancreatitis may rarely be associated with the use of hydrochlorothiazide;
3. gynecomastia has been seen with spironolactone administration;
4. impotence may be associated with use of spironolactone or amiloride;
5. severe watery diarrhea is occasionally seen with ethacrynic acid; and
6. triamterene is a weak folic acid antagonist and may cause megaloblastic anemia in patients with poor nutrition.

Table 11-1 provides a summary of many of the potential complications of diuretics discussed in this chapter.

References

1. 1978: Top 200 drugs. Pharm. Times. April 29, 1979.
2. Schrier, R.W. (editor), Renal and Electrolyte Disorders. 2nd Edition, 1980, Boston, Little, Brown and Company.
3. Narins, R.G., and Gardner, L.B. Simple acid-base disturbances. Med. Clin. No. America. 65:321–346, 1981.
4. Fichman, M.P., Vorherr, H., Kleeman, C.R., and Telfer, N. Diuretic-induced hyponatremia. Ann. Int. Med. 75:853–863, 1971.
5. Nagim, A., Locksley, R., and Arieff, A.I. Thiazide-induced hyponatremia associated with death or neurologic damage in outpatients. Am. J. Med. 70:1163–1168, 1981.
6. Lyons, H., Pinn, V.W., Cortell, S., Cohen, J.J., and Harrington, J.T. Allergic interstitial nephritis causing reversible renal failure in four patients with idiopathic nephrotic syndrome. N. Engl. J. Med. 288:124–128, 1973.
7. Mudge, G.H. Diuretics and other agents employed in the mobilization of edema fluid in: The Pharmacological Basis of Therapeutics. Sixth Edition (editors: A.G. Gilman, L. Goodman and A. Gilman), 1980, New York, Macmillan, pp. 892–915.
8. Physicians' Desk Reference. 37th Edition, 1983, Medical Economics Company.

chapter

12

Diuretic Therapy in Pediatric Patients

Ellis D. Avner, M.D., and Demetrius Ellis, M.D.

As noted in Chapter 1, the rational use of diuretics is predicated upon the recognition of basic physiological principles regarding glomerular and tubular function. Diuretic therapy in older children follows the guidelines presented in the other chapters of this volume for adult patients. However, diuretic usage in neonates and infants must be based upon an understanding of the principles of developmental renal physiology. The process of renal anatomical and functional development, particularly as it relates to the maturation of salt and water handling, is a major determinant of diuretic efficacy and toxicity in the younger pediatric age group. This chapter will therefore discuss: 1) the development of some features of renal glomerular and tubular function and their clinical implications; 2) the clinical pharmacology of diuretic agents used in the pediatric population; and 3) particular diagnostic considerations and applications of diuretic use in children.

Developmental Aspects of Renal Function and Their Clinical Implications

Renal development is a continuous process during which organ function matures in adaptation to changing work requirements. Such development involves the integrated processes of structural and functional maturation in response to the constantly changing hormonal milieu and metabolic demands of the growing organism (1).

Anatomically, the definitive metanephric kidney appears at the fifth week of gestation. Nephrogenesis proceeds in a centrifugal pattern, and the full complement of 1–1.4 million nephrons per kidney has formed by the 35th wk of gestation. The newborn kidney is characterized by physical

TABLE 12-1. Normal Values of Renal Function

Measurement	Premature[a] Newborn	Full-Term Newborn	1–2 wk	6 mo–1 yr	1–3 yr	Adult
GFR (ml/min/1.73 m^2)	14±3	21±4	50±10	77±14	96±22	118±18
Renal Blood Flow (ml/min/1.73 m^2)	40±6	88±4	220±40	352±73	540±118	620±92
TmPAH (mg/min/1.73 m^2)	10±2	16±5	38±8	51±20	66±19	79±12
Maximal Concentrating Ability (mOsm/kg)	480	800	900	1200	1400	1400
Serum Creatinine (mg/dl)	1.3	1.1	0.4	0.2	0.4	0.8–1.5

[a]32–34 wk gestational age.

underdevelopment of proximal tubules relative to glomeruli and the presence of extensive nephron heterogeneity. Because of the centrifugal nature of renal development, the smallest and least mature nephrons are always found in the outermost cortex. This pattern is matched by the distribution of renal blood flow, which is predominantly directed towards corticomedullary nephrons during the first 6 mo of life. During the first 12 postnatal months, nephron growth corrects geographic maturation differences and establishes anatomical glomerulotubular balance through tubular growth. Further increases in renal size involve growth of all parts of the nephron with a major contribution coming from the increased tortuosity of the proximal convoluted tubules and the elongation of the loops of Henle.

Glomerular filtration rate is low at birth, and following a striking postnatal increase during the first 2 wk of life, gradually increases to adult levels by 2–3 yr of age when related to body surface area (Table 12-1) (1). The major factors responsible for the low GFR of infants are a very high level of renal vascular resistance, decreasing the hydrostatic pressure of ultrafiltration ($\overline{P}_{uf}$), and a low total surface area available for filtration (S). The GFR of premature infants (less than 34 wk gestational age) is even lower than that of term infants, and increases at a slower rate postnatally. In concert with changes in GFR, sodium excretory capacity also undergoes maturation during the first postnatal years (2). Pre-term infants have an imbalance between glomerular and tubular function with regard to the capacity for sodium reabsorption. This glomerulotubular imbalance is a function of decreased proximal tubular sodium reabsorption due to structural immaturity and incomplete development of tubular transport enzyme systems as well as partial distal nephron unresponsiveness to high circulating levels of mineralocorticoids. The high fractional sodium excretion in pre-term newborns can lead to negative sodium balance and symptomatic hyponatremia if sodium intake does not match urinary losses. Full-term newborns have a low basal sodium excretion and in contrast to premature infants, are able to retain sodium when in negative salt balance. In full-term newborns, increases in GFR and filtered sodium load are matched by increases in proximal tubular sodium reabsorption as the basolateral surface of the proximal tubule undergoes development. Although proximal sodium reabsorption lags behind glomerular filtration rate during the first year of life in such infants, exaggerated sodium loss does not occur because of enhanced reabsorption of sodium in the distal convoluted tubule (2). Such enhanced transport of sodium occurs under the stimulation of a high plasma concentration of aldosterone. Positive sodium balance is essential to growth because the accretion of body tissue, particularly bone, requires the retention of sodium. A well-established characteristic of sodium metabolism in both premature and term infants is a limited ability to excrete a sodium load (3). This sodium retention is primarily due to enhanced sodium reabsorption in the distal convoluted tubule under the control of aldosterone, although the low GFR and anatomical predominance of juxtamedullary to superficial nephrons may also play a role.

The tubular transport system for excretion of endogenous and exogenous organic acids is poorly developed in both premature and term newborns (1). The tubular transport of such organic acids, represented by PAH secretion (TmPAH), increases progressively with age, and reaches adult levels by 1–3 yr (Table 12-1). Tubular excretion of weak acids is limited by: 1) low GFR, 2) anatomical immaturity leading to low tubular secretory surface area and poor access of organic acid to tubular transporting membrane, 3) a low number of transporting sites per unit of tubular surface area, and 4) incomplete development of metabolic processes providing energy for acid transport. In addition to immaturity of tubular organic acid excretion, young children demonstrate incomplete renal acid-base homeostasis. Newborns and infants have lower levels of plasma pH and bicarbonate concentration than adults. This phenomenon is related to incomplete renal proximal tubular bicarbonate reabsorption, impaired renal distal tubular excretion of titratable acid due to lack of urinary buffers, and incomplete development of distal tubular ammonia production. Although the precise time course for maturation of each of these functions has not been established for humans, it appears that renal acid-base homeostatic mechanisms reach adult capabilities by 2 yr of age.

In both pre-term and term infants, a water load cannot be excreted as well as in the adult (4). The ability to respond to a water load improves rapidly during the first few weeks of life, reaching adult capabilities by 3–5 wk postnatally. Under certain conditions, newborn infants can dilute their urine to the same degree as can adults (50 mOsm/kg). It therefore appears that a primary factor in the incomplete response to water loading is the decreased fluid load presented to diluting segments of the nephron secondary to a low GFR. In contrast to diluting capacity, the concentrating capacity of premature and full-term infants is low at birth and continues to increase during the first year of life to approach adult levels at approximately 2 yr of age (Table 12-1). This concentrating defect appears to be a consequence of the incomplete development of several factors responsible for the hypertonicity of the inner medulla which is required for maximal concentration. Incomplete reabsorption of sodium in the water-impermeable ascending loop of Henle, decreased urea accumulation in the medulla and the papilla, and the short length of the medullary loops of Henle and the collecting ducts all impair maximal concentration in the neonate and infant. Further, an additional factor contributing to impaired concentrating ability is suggested by experimental studies which indicate that the collecting duct cells of immature nephrons are less sensitive to the effect of ADH than those of the mature nephron.

The principles of edema formation in infants and children are generally the same as those described for adults (Chapter 1). However, the clinical effectiveness of diuretics in the management of edema is based on the unique nature of glomerular and tubular function present at different stages of development (5). The low GFR of premature infants limits the effectiveness of thiazide diuretics. Furosemide, ethacrynic acid, or bumetanide must be used in the treatment of salt and water retention secondary to any primary disease process in this age group. An important consideration of diuretic therapy in the premature infant is the limited ability of the proximal tubule to reabsorb sodium even under conditions of negative salt balance, thus increasing the risk of diuretic-induced contraction of ECF volume. Any such decrease in ECF volume, superimposed upon the low GFR already present at this stage of renal development, can lead to the development of significant volume depletion, severe azotemia, and acute renal failure. In full-term infants and children during the first yr of life, salt and water retention secondary to any primary disease process is further complicated by the enhanced activity of the renin-angiotensin-aldosterone axis and consequent avid distal tubular sodium reabsorption. The therapy of all edema-forming states in this age group should include the early use of diuretic agents whose sites of action are the late portion of the distal convolution and the collecting duct such as spironolactone and triamterene (Appendix 2). Such agents, which are effective in blocking sodium reabsorption at distal nephron sites, may have increased diuretic and natriuretic potency during the first 2 yr of life. However, despite their utility, such distally acting agents, particularly when used alone, may precipitate a hyperkalemic metabolic acidosis because of the low underlying GFR present during this period (Chapter 11).

The immaturity of tubular organic acid transport in young children alters the excretion of diuretics and other drugs which are normally removed by this system. Agents requiring dosage adjustments because of renal immaturity of this elimination pathway include acetazolamide, chlorothiazide, ethacrynic acid, and furosemide (Table 12-2). The failure to recognize this feature of tubular immaturity in young children may lead to drug accumulation and increased risks of drug-related toxicity. The incomplete development of renal mechanisms for maintaining acid-base homeostasis has additional clinical implications regarding diuretic usage in young infants. Carbonic anhydrase inhibitors, such as acetazolamide, carry a significant risk of inducing metabolic acidosis in this setting. Such agents are therefore contraindicated in young infants. Finally, the impaired renal concentrating ability of young children's kidneys also has implications with regard to diuretic usage. Agents which affect the concentrating mechanism, such as furosemide and other loop agents (see Appendix 1), can lower maximal osmolar excretion below the demands created by normal dietary intake and metabolism. This may result in serum hyperosmolarity with its attendant hazards if renal solute load is not decreased by dietary changes.

Clinical Pharmacology

Despite the extensive use of diuretics in the pediatric population over the last two decades, there is a paucity of well-controlled studies on the effectiveness and toxicity of various diuretic regimens in children. There are significant age-related variations in the bioavailability, volume of distribution, biotransformation, and elimination of most classes of drugs. However, clinical usage of diuretics in the pediatric age group has largely been based on data extrapolated from pharmacological studies in adults. Although there are a large number of diuretic agents available for use in children, not all are of value, and several should be used under only very specific conditions (6). The guidelines for the use of diuretics in children presented in Table 12-2 are based upon limited studies in pediatric patients, pharmacological data generated in adult patients, as well as the known pharmacology of diuretic agents and the principles of developmental physiology and pharmacology. This table summarizes currently available data on appropriate dosage regimens for diuretic use in the pediatric population and denotes unusual features and toxicity of various diuretic regimens.

TABLE 12-2. Clinical Use of Diuretic Agents in Infants and Children[a]

Drug and Dosage	Uses	Special Considerations
Furosemide (Lasix)		
1 mg/kg/dose IV or PO. dose of 4 mg/kg/IV mg/kg/day in premature infants. Single dose of 4/mg/kg/IV in oliguric children with acute renal failure and normal or high central venous pressure.	Edema due to congestive heart failure, nephrosis, or hepatic failure; hypertension; to enhance the excretion of calcium, barbiturates, uric acid, halides and salicylates; SIADH.	Low renal clearance and/or decreased metabolism causes slow elimination in newborns of various gestational ages causing ototoxicity, prolonged diuretic and saliuretic effects. Avoid in infants with plasma bilirubin ≥10 mg/dl since drug can cause extensive displacement of bilirubin from albumin and increase risk of kernicterus. Hypercalciuria can lead to renal stones and nephrocalcinosis in infants receiving ≥2 mg/kg/day for more than 12 days. This may be prevented by adding chlorothiazide.
Ethacrynic acid (Edecrin)		
0.5–1.0 mg/kg/dose IV; 1–2 mg/kg/day PO in 3 doses.	Same as for furosemide. Use in patients whose diuresis becomes refractory to furosemide or patients with hypersensitivity to furosemide.	Same as for furosemide.
Bumetanide (Bumex)		
Dose not determined in children. ? 0.25–0.5 mg/dose IV: ? 0.5–1.0 mg/dose PO.	Edematous states in place of furosemide or when patients may become refractory to furosemide.	Not evaluated in infants and children. 1 mg bumetanide is ≃40 mg furosemide. More efficient intestinal absorption than furosemide and may be more effective than furosemide in patients with low GFR or acid-base disturbances. Same considerations as for furosemide and ethacrynic acid in terms of protein binding and side-effects.
Chlorothiazide (Diuril)		
20–40 mg/kg/day PO in 2 doses.	Hypertension; edema; hypercalciuria; nephrogenic or pituitary diabetes insipidus.	At equipotent doses, it displaces more bilirubin from albumin than does furosemide. Must be used in conjunction with salt restriction to be effective in patients with diabetes insipidus.
Hydrochlorothiazide (Hydrodiuril)		
2–3.5 mg/kg/day PO in 1–2 doses.	Same as for chlorothiazide.	Same as for chlorothiazide.

TABLE 12-2 *(continued)*

Drug and Dosage	Uses	Special Considerations
Spironolactone (Aldactone) 1–2 mg/kg/day PO in 2 doses.	Adjunct to kaliuretic drugs in states of hyperaldosteronism such as congestive heart failure, hepatic cirrhosis, and nephrotic syndrome.	By enhancing natriuretic response of diuretics acting in a more proximal region of the renal tubule, it may potentiate diuresis while neutralizing kaliuresis. Combined with chlorothiazide, it is very effective in infants with congestive heart failure associated with respiratory distress syndrome and patent ductus arteriosus. In patients with localized edema (e.g., ascites) or those with 1° or 2° hyperaldosteronism, start treatment with this drug alone, and add furosemide or a thiazide diuretic only if needed.
Metolazone (Zaroxolyn, Diulo) 0.5–2.5 mg/day PO in 1–2 doses.	Adjunct to management of hypertension and edematous states.	Combined with furosemide, may be particularly effective in edema states in which urine flow is reduced such as chronic congestive heart failure in infants. Avoid use in advanced renal failure.
Aminophylline	Not used as a diuretic. Used in treatment of asthma and apneic spells.	As with corticosteroids, aminophylline can increase GFR and can cause natriuresis and secondary diuresis, volume contraction and hyponatremia, especially in premature infants.
Mannitol 0.2 gm/kg IV over 3–5 min if oliguria is present. 1.5–2.0 gm/kg IV as 20% soln. if urine flow is preserved.	Test dose in oliguric acute renal failure. Use early in course of myoglobinuria, hemoglobinuria or hyperuricemic acute renal failure.	If unable to be excreted, risks for hyperosmolarity and secondary problems of intraventricular hemorrhage or pulmonary edema are particularly high in newborns and premature infants.

[a]Mechanism of action and side-effects other than those discussed under Special Considerations are the same as for adults (see Chapter 11 and Appendix II). Note that elimination of all of the above diuretics is primarily renal. Therefore, repetitive use of these drugs is contraindicated in oliguric children. Diuretic secretion into breast milk or transplacental passage of these drugs is not known to cause significant diuresis, volume depletion, electrolyte imbalance, hematologic abnormalities, or other untoward effects in young infants, but data are scant.

Diagnostic Considerations and Applications of Diuretic Use in Children

Similar to their use in adult patients, diuretics are utilized in children to treat generalized edema secondary to congestive heart failure, nephrotic syndrome, renal insufficiency, or hepatic cirrhosis (5). In addition, diuretics are also clinically used in the treatment of conditions not associated with the formation of generalized edema which include hypertension, hypercalcemia, hypercalciuria, hydrocephalus, cerebral edema, exogenous poisoning, the syndrome of inappropriate anti-diuretic hormone secretion (SIADH), diabetes insipidus, and hypokalemic periodic paralysis. The pathophysiology and differential diagnosis of edema-forming states and the clinical indications for diuretic use are similar in adults and children, and are extensively covered in the other chapters of this volume. However, there are two particular situations which are encountered only in the pediatric population and require further discussion: 1) the diagnosis and treatment of edema in the newborn and young infant; and 2) the clinical use of diuretics in infants with the respiratory distress syndrome.

Edema in the Newborn and Young Infant

As noted in Chapter 1, edema is the clinical expression of expansion of the interstitial compartment of the extracellular fluid (ECF) volume. This expansion may occur from positive sodium and water balance leading to overall ECF expansion, or enhanced transfer of fluid into the interstitial compartment due to alterations in Starling forces across capillary membranes. Both of these factors are of major importance in the pathogenesis of edema formation in the newborn or young infant, which may be associated with a number of conditions (Table 12-3) (7). Edema may occur in the newborn period unrelated to any known pathological condition, and is thus termed idiopathic. This idiopathic edema, more common in

TABLE 12-3. Conditions Associated with Edema in Newborns and Infants

Idiopathic edema of the newborn
Hypoxia in utero
Hydrops fetalis
Vitamin E deficiency
Angioneurotic edema
Lymphedema
Turner's syndrome
Congenital heart disease
Congenital renal disease

premature infants and those born by cesarean section, is not present at birth but develops within the first 24 hr of life. In some instances, the edema has been noted before the infant has received oral fluids, and at a time when body weight has decreased from birth weight. Balance studies indicate that the edematous state is primarily due to shifts of fluid from the intracellular to the extracellular space and from the intravascular to the interstitial compartment without expansion of total body sodium or water. The mechanism of such shifting, which opposes the normal readjustment of body composition occurring in transition from intra to extra-uterine existence, is unknown. Edema in this syndrome spontaneously resolves by the end of the second postnatal week without dietary sodium restriction or diuretic therapy.

Edema in the newborn has also been associated with hypoxia in-utero. Such intrauterine hypoxia causes an abnormal total body fluid shift from the maternal to fetal circulation, and also produces increased vascular permeability in the newborn. The asphyxiated newborn therefore has an expanded ECF volume, increased movement of fluid from the intravascular to interstitial fluid compartments because of abnormal capillary membranes, and decreased effective arterial plasma volume leading to renal mechanisms for further salt and water retention. Therapy of edema in such infants involves the judicious use of colloid-containing intravenous solutions to maintain a normal serum colloid osmotic pressure and maximize effective arterial plasma volume. Diuretics are only indicated if intravascular volume support leads to the development of pulmonary or cardiac failure.

Hydrops fetalis refers to excessive accumulation of fluid by the fetus leading to anasarca in the newborn. Three mechanisms are generally operative in producing hydrops fetalis: 1) decreased fetal hepatic albumin synthesis with resultant hypoalbuminemia and low plasma colloid osmotic pressure; 2) chronic intrauterine high output heart failure secondary to anemia; and 3) abnormal fluid redistribution between the intravascular and interstitial spaces secondary to a diffuse increase in capillary permeability caused by chronic anemia and tissue hypoxia. Although traditionally described as a consequence of Rh hemolytic disease of the newborn, hydrops fetalis may be associated with a number of pathological conditions operative during intrauterine life which include: other hemolytic anemias; congestive heart failure secondary to arrhythmias or congenital heart disease; vascular malformations of fetal membranes, liver, or brain; intrauterine vascular accidents; congenital infections; pulmonary malformations; neuroblastoma or tuberous sclerosis; congenital nephrosis; and syndromes of multiple organ malformation including the Trisomy E syndrome. Management of the infant with hydrops includes initial resuscitation and subsequent stabilization. In the delivery room, severe respiratory depression, ascites, pleural effusions, and pulmonary edema may be present and require intubation, positive pressure ventilation, abdominal paracentesis, and thoracentesis. Intravascular volume depletion and low serum colloid osmotic pressure are treated with vigorous colloid and blood replacement. Exchange transfusion is utilized in hemolytic anemias. Pulmonary edema is optimally managed by continuous positive airway pressure and judicious use of furosemide and digitalis once circulating volume is adequate. Management of the generalized body edema is approached by moderate fluid restriction (60–80 ml/kg/day) and sodium restriction (1–2 mEq/kg/day) after initial stabilization. Spontaneous diuresis usually ensues between 3–6 days following birth and results in a maximal weight loss by 14 days of age. The spontaneous diuresis may be brisk with weight decreasing from 20 to 45 percent of birthweight, and a contraction metabolic alkalosis may develop if ECF volume is not supported.

Other unusual conditions associated with generalized edema in infants include Vitamin E deficiency, angioneurotic edema, lymphedema, and Turner's syndrome. In these conditions, abnormal capillary permeability or generalized lymphatic abnormalities alter the effective balance of Starling forces. Diuretics are not indicated in such conditions, and therapy is directed at maximizing colloid osmotic pressure, and, if possible, specific therapy of the underlying condition. Edema may also be seen in newborns with congenital heart disease and congestive heart failure. The principles of treatment of congestive heart failure include appropriate diuretic and inotropic therapy as discussed in Chapter 4, in addition to anatomical correction of structural anomalies when possible. Renal failure secondary to congenital anomalies or nephrotic syndrome may also be associated with edema in infancy. The principles of management of these conditions are in general the same as their adult counterparts (Chapters 2 and 8).

Diuretic Use in Hyaline Membrane Disease

Hyaline membrane disease (HMD) is the most common cause of respiratory distress during the first days of life and occurs in approximately one percent of all newborns. The major factor that predisposes newborns to the development of HMD is prematurity; however, the disease is also more common in infants born by cesarean section, infants of diabetic mothers, and infants who suffer from perinatal asphyxia. The disease is due to inadequate production of pulmonary surfactant, which raises the surface tension within pulmonary alveoli and results in respiratory units which inflate with difficulty and do not remain gas filled between respiratory efforts. The clinical manifestation of this abnormality is progressive atelectasis which leads to increasingly labored breathing during the first hours of life. Progressive ventilation-perfusion mismatching and alveolar hypoventilation cause progressive cyanosis and hypercarbia. A major factor in the progression of severe HMD is the development of pulmonary interstitial and alveolar edema which further decreases surfactant production and promotes hypoxia. In addition, 30 to 40 percent of infants with HMD will develop the persistence of a patent ductus arteriosus, which further exacerbates pulmonary edema by causing increased pulmonary blood flow and an increase in pulmonary venous capillary pressure secondary to volume overload and congestive heart failure. The basic management of HMD is aggressive respiratory support by continuous positive airway pressure or mechanical ventilation. However, diuretics, particularly furosemide, have been used extensively in the fluid and metabolic management of infants with HMD (8). The rationale for furosemide use in HMD has been based on a number of factors. First, it has been reasoned that the overall negative sodium and water balance induced by the drug would decrease pulmonary interstitial and alveolar edema, and therefore improve surfactant development and oxygenation. Second, in infants with congestive heart failure secondary to a patent ductus arteriosus, a diuretic-induced decrease in ECF volume would decrease left atrial pressure, pulmonary blood flow, and the increase in pulmonary venous capillary pressures favoring the development of interstitial pulmonary edema. Thirdly, studies have revealed that the use of furosemide in infants with this syndrome has led to a decrease in systemic venous pressures and increases in serum colloid osmotic pressure, which is independent of its diuretic action and presumably related to the stimulation of renal prostaglandin synthesis. Finally, it has been a long-standing clinical observation that infants who survive HMD often have a large spontaneous diuresis which heralds a dramatic improvement in respiratory function. Therefore, it has been reasoned that the use of furosemide to artificially promote such a natriuresis and diuresis might similarly improve ventilatory function by a number of different mechanisms. Because of these considerations, it has been estimated that greater than 50 percent of infants with severe respiratory distress syndrome are treated with furosemide during their course.

Despite the rationale for furosemide use in HMD, current data suggest that the use of this agent may have limited value in this syndrome. The spontaneous diuresis which presages recovery in the natural history of HMD has been related to decreasing renal production of prostacyclin (PGI_2). As PGI_2 increases vascular permeability and stimulates renin release, a decrease in its synthesis is associated with increased vascular integrity, increased colloid osmotic pressure, mobilization of interstitial fluid, decreased angiotensin-mediated changes in renal blood flow, and a subsequent rise in urine output with improvement in ventilation. Thus, spontaneous recovery from HMD is not related to simple diuresis per se, but rather reflects the multiple systemic actions of hormonal and vasoactive factors to improve vascular integrity, decrease pulmonary fluid accumulation, and improve effective arterial plasma volume. In this regard, it has been noted previously that furosemide, in an effect independent of its diuretic action, increases the renal production of PGI_2 and prostaglandin E_2 (PGE_2). Its use in HMD might therefore adversely affect the balance of hormonal factors known to mediate improvement in overall systemic hemodynamics in this syndrome. Further (and somewhat paradoxically, since furosemide has traditionally been used to treat heart failure in the newborn population), furosemide-induced increases in renal prostaglandin E_1 synthesis appear to promote the development of a patent ductus arteriosus with its deleterious effects on the course of HMD.

As noted previously, thiazide diuretics have not been clinically useful in the treatment of positive sodium and water balance in young infants. Further, there are no studies on the pharmacological effect of ethacrynic acid or bumetanide in newborn infants. Therefore, it is recommended that the use of furosemide in neonates with HMD be restricted to those instances where severe ECF volume overload mandates diuretic therapy. In such instances, the use of furosemide may require concomitant therapy with prostaglandin synthetase inhibitors or surgical ligation of a patent ductus arteriosus. The limited clinical usefulness of furosemide in infants with HMD, and its effects on bilirubin binding and the incidence of nephrolithiasis in young infants (Table 12-2) are striking examples of the need to consider the principles of developmental renal physiology and pharmacology in the use of diuretics in young infants.

References

1. Spitzer, A. Renal physiology and functional development, Chapter 2, In: Pediatric Kidney Disease, 1978 (editor: C.M. Edelmann, Jr.), Boston, Little Brown and Co., pp. 25–127.
2. Spitzer, A. The role of the kidney in sodium homeostasis during maturation. Kidney Int. 21:539–545, 1982.
3. Rodriquez-Soriano, R., Vallo, A., Castillo, G., and Oliveros, R. Renal handling of water and sodium in infancy and childhood: a study using clearance methods during hypotonic saline diuresis. Kidney Int. 20:700–704, 1981.
4. Aperia, A., and Zelterström, R. Renal control of fluid homeostasis in the newborn infant. Clin. Perinatol. 9:523–533, 1982.
5. Loggie, J.M.H., Kleinman, L.I., and Van Maanen, E.F. Renal function and diuretic therapy in infants and children. J. Pediatr. 86:485–496, 657–669, 825–832, 1975.
6. Bailie, M.D., Linshaw, M.A., and Stygles, V.G. Diuretic pharmacology in infants and children. Pediatr. Clin. North Am. 28:217–230, 1981.
7. Lewy, J.E. Diuretics in infancy. Contrib. Nephrol. 27:33–44, 1981.
8. Green, T.P. The use of diuretics in infants with the respiratory distress syndrome. Semin. Perinatol. 6:172–180, 1982.

chapter

13

Diuretic Drug Interactions with Other Agents

Patricia D. Kroboth, Ph. D.

Two drugs administered concurrently may result in an increase, a decrease, or no change in the observed effect of one or both drugs. A change in drug effect can be caused by a pharmacokinetic interaction which occurs when one drug affects the absorption, distribution, metabolism or excretion pattern of another drug. The result is generally a change in either duration or quantity of drug available for pharmacologic effect, with a corresponding change in the magnitude or duration of that effect. Alternatively, an interaction can be pharmacodynamic in nature, with modification of the observed drug effect resulting from the action of two drugs on effector cells.

Because of differing diuretic mechanisms and sites of action, various diuretic-drug combinations may not elicit the same clinical response. There are over 100 reports of interactions between diuretic medications and other agents. However, not all of the interactions are well documented, nor are all of the interactions of clinical significance. In this chapter, interactions with commonly used drugs which have been well documented or which have potentially severe clinical consequences are discussed. A summary of these appears in Table 13-1, which also includes interactions that have been described in only a few patients or are of limited significance because of infrequent use of the medication.

Digoxin

Description and summary. Both pharmacodynamic and pharmacokinetic interactions have been described.

1. *Decreased digoxin inotropy.* Digoxin induced inotropy is abolished by amiloride and inhibited to a lesser extent by spironolactone (1). This

TABLE 13-1. Interactions Between Diuretics and Other Agents

Diuretic Agent	Drug	Interaction	Type of Report	Comment	References
Furosemide	Acetylsalicyclic acid	Decreased natriuresis but protection from salicylate-induced decrease in renal function	Study in cirrhotic patients with ascites	See text	11
Furosemide	Aminoglycosides	1. Suggestion of enhanced ototoxicity in patients receiving both		Poor documentation	19, p. 78
		2. 57% decrease in gentamicin clearance and 33% increase in plasma concentration at 90 min	Study in patients	Each agent independently causes ototoxicity	20
Furosemide	Chloral hydrate	Diaphoresis, variable blood pressure after IV furosemide when chloral hydrate administered in previous 24 hr	Case report and retrospective study	See text	14,15
Furosemide	Cisplatin	Possible cisplatin nephrotoxicity	Letter reporting a single case	Use caution when altering renal hemodynamics within a few hours following cisplatin	21
Furosemide	Clofibrate	Muscle stiffness and pain with marked diuresis in 6 patients	Report of 6 cases	Use caution in prescribing the combination. Limit clofibrate dose to 500 mg for each 1 g albumin/100 ml	22

Furosemide	Lithium	Lithium toxicity when furosemide is added	Studies in patients and volunteers	See text	4
Furosemide	Phenytoin	Decrease of approximately 50% in diuretic response	2 studies in patients and in normal volunteers	Larger doses of furosemide may be required	23
Furosemide	Probenecid	Delayed natriuresis; overall response may be increased or decreased, depending on diuretic dose	Studies in normal volunteers	Probably not a clinically significant interaction. No precautions necessary	24
Furosemide	Propranolol	1. Enhanced β-blockade 2. Reports of both increased and decreased propranolol clearance	Studies in normal volunteers	Probably not a clinically significant interaction	25
Furosemide, bumetanide	Prostaglandin synthetase inhibitors	Decreased diuretic and hypotensive effects	Studies in patients and normal volunteers	See text	8,9
Furosemide	Theophylline	Increased theophylline concentrations (0.5–5.5 μg/ml). No toxicity observed	Study in 10 patients	Monitor theophylline concentrations	26
Furosemide	Tubocurare	Enhancement of neuromuscular blockade	Case report in 3 patients	Use caution when administering these agents together	19, p. 393
Ethacrynic acid	Aminoglycosides	Additive ototoxicity demonstrated with kanamycin, streptomycin, neomycin	Case reports, studies with small numbers of patients	Combination should be avoided	19, p. 77
Ethacrynic acid	Warfarin	Increased prothrombin time	Single case report	Avoid combination, or monitor prothrombin time carefully; see text	16

(continued on next page)

TABLE 13-1 *(continued)*

Diuretic Agent	Drug	Interaction	Type of Report	Comment	References
Thiazides	Allopurinol	Severe hypersensitivity reaction in patients with renal disease taking both drugs	Case report, retrospective study	Caution suggested regarding combined use in patients with abnormal renal function	27,28
Chlorthiazide	Colestipol, cholestyramine	Decreased absorption of chlorthiazide when administration separated by 1 hr	Study in 10 patients	Do not give simultaneously; separate doses by a minimum of 2 hr	29
Thiazides, ethacrynic acid, furosemide	Corticosteroids with mineralocorticoid effect	Excessive potassium depletion		Maintain adequate potassium supplementation	19, p. 437
Thiazides	Cyclophosphamide-methotrexate fluorouracil	Augmentation of granulocytopenia in 14 women with breast cancer	Crossover design study in patients	See text	13
Thiazides, chlorthalidone, ethacrynic acid	Hypoglycemic agents	Hyperglycemic effects can antagonize diabetic control	Studies in patients	Some patients may need an increase in hypoglycemic agent dosage	19, p. 343
Hydrochlorothiazide	Propantheline	Delayed but increased absorption of hydrochlorothiazide	Study in 6 normal volunteers	Clinical significance unknown, but probably minimal	19, p. 460
Thiazides	Prostaglandin synthetase inhibitors	Decreased diuretic and hypotensive effects	Studies in patients and normal volunteers	See text	7,9

Spironolactone	Warfarin	Decreased effect of warfarin	Study in 9 normal volunteers	Increased warfarin dose may be needed; caution when starting, stopping spironolactone	17
Triamterene	Indomethacin	Acute renal failure in 2 of 4 subjects taking combination	Study of 4 normal volunteers	Do not use combination; see text	12
Acetazolamide, spirono-lactone, triamterene	Lithium	Possibility of increased lithium excretion	Studies in volunteers and 2 patients	Inconclusive evidence; monitor lithium concentrations and response when adding any diuretic	19, p. 346
Acetazolamide	Methadone	Alkalinization of urine causes decreased renal excretion of methadone, which is not ionized at alkaline pH	Study in patients	Effect on clinical response unknown. May need to adjust methadone dose downward	30
Acetazolamide	Quinidine	Alkalinization of urine causes increased tubular reabsorp-tion of quinidine	Study in normal volunteers	Quinidine concentrations and response should be monitored when acetazo-lamide or other urinary alkalinizers are added or withdrawn.	19, p. 66
Acetazolamide	Radionuclide used for cisternogram	Abnormal cisternogram possibly due to inhibition of CSF formation	Case report	Discontinue acetazolamide 2 or 3 days prior to study; See text	18

information is based on studies in normal volunteers and suggests a potential pharmacodynamic interaction between these agents and digoxin. This effect of spironolactone has also been demonstrated in patients with congestive heart failure (2). The mechanism for this is unknown. Triamterene, thiazides and loop diuretics do not share in this effect.

2. *Decreased digoxin clearance.* Digoxin total body clearance is decreased 35% by spironolactone and 20% by triamterene, but is unaffected by amiloride. Spironolactone's effect is entirely due to reduced renal tubular secretion of digoxin. Triamterene does not change renal tubular digoxin secretion, while amiloride enhances it; both reduce extrarenal clearance (1). Although a transient increase in digoxin excretion may be observed during a brisk furosemide diuresis, the effect on digoxin stores is probably negligible (3).
3. *Enhanced digoxin effects/toxicity.* Depletion of potassium enhances digoxin effects. Since all diuretics except "potassium sparing" agents cause potassium loss, potassium supplementation may be needed in digitalized patients.

Conclusions and management. Spironolactone and especially amiloride should be avoided as first line agents when digoxin is prescribed for its inotropic effect. Decreased digoxin inotropy is not seen with triamterene and has not been described with thiazides or loop diuretics. These non-interacting diuretics are preferred alternatives.

When triamterene or spironolactone is added to digoxin therapy, plasma digoxin concentrations should be monitored to avoid toxicity due to the decrease in total body digoxin clearance.

Lithium

Description and summary. Thiazides cause retention of lithium with a resultant increase in serum lithium concentration and risk of toxicity. Lithium is excreted by the kidney, with reabsorption occurring in the proximal tubule. Although conflicting results have been reported, it is thought that any diuretic or treatment (low sodium diet) which depletes sodium will increase proximal reabsorption of both sodium and lithium. The interaction may not be limited to effects on lithium excretion, however. An enhanced response to lithium at equivalent serum concentrations, following a reduction in lithium dose, has been reported when therapy included thiazides or a low sodium diet (4).

Lithium toxicity can result if a thiazide is added to the medication regimen of a patient with therapeutic lithium concentrations. This same phenomenon may be observed with loop diuretics.

Conclusions and management. The lithium dose should be decreased by approximately 50% when adding thiazides, chlorthalidone or loop diuretics (5). Lithium concentrations and response should be carefully monitored and the dose titrated to maintain therapeutic effect.

Prostaglandin Synthetase Inhibitors (PGSI)

Prostaglandins are synthesized on demand from arachidonic acid by essentially all tissues. In the kidney, prostaglandins appear to have a role in the regulation of intrarenal hemodynamics and glomerular filtration. This is especially true in patients with renal disease and hypoperfusion states. Prostaglandins E_2, D_2, and I_2 reduce renal vascular resistance and increase renal blood flow. Indomethacin, the PGSI which has been studied most extensively, has been found to impair the synthesis of prostaglandins in response to hemorrhage, hypotension and angiotensin II (6). Other PGSI's, including salicylates, ibuprofen, fenoprofen, naproxen, mefanamic acid and tolmetin, appear to have similar types of effects in the kidney. The exception is sulindac, which inhibits only extrarenal prostaglandin synthesis (7). Furosemide, ethacrynic acid and bumetanide, but not thiazide diuretics, appear to inhibit prostaglandin breakdown. Their natriuretic effects, however, are not entirely due to their effects on prostaglandins (6). Because of differences in diuretic and PGSI mechanisms and potency, various diuretic-PGSI combinations can be expected to have different clinical effects.

Description and summary. Three types of effects have been reported as the result of interactions between PGSI's and diuretics: 1) reduced hypotensive effects; 2) reduced diuretic effectiveness/protection from PGSI induced decrease in renal function; and 3) acute renal failure. These effects are discussed separately.

1. *Reduced hypotensive effects.* Addition of indomethacin to regimens of hypertensive patients has resulted in decreased blood pressure control. This effect has been noted with furosemide (8) and thiazides (7, 9). The mechanism by which indomethacin interferes with blood pressure lowering effects is unknown. Based on information from one study (7), sulindac does not share in this blunting of anti-hypertensive effect.
2. *Reduced diuretic effectiveness/protection from decreased renal function.* It appears that the degree of antagonism between PGSI's and diuretics depends on the state of sodium balance, the renin-angiotensin axis and renal hemodynamics. PGSI's have been reported to blunt natriuresis and diuresis in some studies, but not in others. Patients

with essential hypertension, nephrotic syndrome and impaired kidney function show decreased response to diuretics when a PGSI is added (10), while variable responses have been noted in normal subjects. This decrease in natriuresis and diuresis has also been noted in cirrhotic patients with ascites when a salicylic acid derivative was administered prior to furosemide. As a positive effect of this interaction, furosemide protected patients from salicylate-induced renal insufficiency which was observed when salicylate was administered alone (11).

Neither this effect nor the attenuation of blood pressure control appears to be due to changes in absorption or elimination patterns of diuretics.

3. *Acute renal failure.* Two of four normal subjects developed acute renal failure when given a combination of triamterene and indomethacin (12). Neither triamterene nor indomethacin alone produced changes in renal function, although urinary PGE_2 excretion was increased with triamterene and decreased by indomethacin. Effects on PGE_2 were more marked in the subjects who developed renal failure. The reason for the toxicity of this particular combination is unclear.

Conclusions and management. Not every person who receives the combination of triamterene and indomethacin will develop toxicity. Because of the severity of the toxicity and availability of suitable alternatives, triamterene and indomethacin should not be administered concurrently.

Although not all PGSI's have been evaluated, certainly the potential for an interaction between any diuretic and any PGSI exists. The extent and clinical significance of the interaction will depend on the patient's hemodynamic status as well as the type of PGSI and diuretic prescribed. Alternatives include discontinuing the PGSI, using a PGSI with little intrarenal prostaglandin effect, such as sulindac, or using higher doses of diuretic.

Cyclophosphamide-Methotrexate-Fluorouracil (CMF)

Diuretics Implicated—Thiazides

Description and summary. Augmentation of granulocytopenia was observed in 14 women with breast cancer who received CMF along with a thiazide for hypertension (13). After a minimum of three cycles, the thiazide was replaced with either propranolol or reserpine. Both mean granulocyte count and nadir were significantly higher during cycles without thiazides. The mechanism is unknown.

Conclusion and management. Although the information available is from only one study, it seems that thiazides should be used with caution in women undergoing treatment with CMF. Whether this represents an interaction between thiazides and a single agent in this regimen is unclear.

Chloral Hydrate

Diuretic Implicated—Furosemide

Description and summary. Diaphoresis, weakness, nausea, hot flashes and blood pressure variability have been reported immediately following an IV dose of furosemide when chloral hydrate had been administered as a nocturnal sedative within the previous 24 hr (14, 15). One report documents the reaction in a single patient, and states that six other patients experienced similar episodes (14). Of 43 patients in a retrospective study who received the combination, there were 1 definite and 2 probable reactions (15). No patient in any of three control groups (total patients: 125) experienced the reaction. The mechanism is unknown.

Conclusions and management. This appears to be a relatively uncommon reaction which does not occur in every patient who receives the combination. However, because of the severity of the reaction and the availability of several sedative-hypnotic benzodiazepines which have not been implicated in the interaction, the combination of chloral hydrate and intravenous furosemide should probably be avoided.

Warfarin

Diuretics Interacting—Ethacrynic Acid and Spironolactone

Description and summary. Administration of ethacrynic acid on two separate occasions to a single patient taking warfarin resulted in an increase in prothrombin time (16). An *in vitro* binding study supports the hypothesis that ethacrynic acid decreases the protein binding of warfarin.

In a study of a spironotactone-warfarin interaction in normal volunteers, spironolactone decreased the effect of warfarin (17).

Conclusions and management. The data on warfarin interactions with ethacrynic acid and spironolactone are limited. However, warfarin interactions with other diuretics have not been described. Use of diuretics other than ethacrynic acid and spironolactone is recommended for patients taking warfarin. If one of the agents must be used in a patient taking warfarin, the prothrombin time should be followed carefully.

Radionuclide Used in Cisternogram

Diuretic Interacting—Acetazolamide

Description and summary. Cisternogram consistent with normal-pressure hydrocephalus was observed in a patient taking acetazolamide and reverted to normal within five days of discontinuing the medication (17). The abnormal cisternogram was thought to be due to carbonic anhydrase inhibition with subsequent reduction in cerebrospinal fluid formation. The result was altered CSF flow with net reflux of tracer into the ventricular system.

Conclusions and management. Despite the fact that the information is limited to one case report, acetazolamide should be discontinued two to three days prior to performing a cisternogram.

Potassium Preparations

Diuretics Interacting—Amiloride, Spironolactone, and Triamterene

Descriptions and summary. Simultaneous administration can result in excessively high potassium concentrations because of an inability to effectively excrete potassium in the presence of these agents. This is especially true in patients with reduced renal function.

Conclusions and management. Concurrent administration should be avoided. If potassium supplements and a diuretic of this type are used together to increase potassium, serum electrolytes should be monitored very closely to prevent dangerously high potassium concentrations and fatal arrhythmias.

References

1. Waldorff, S., Hansen, P.B., Egeblad, H., Berning, J., Buch, J., Kjaergard, H., and Steiness, E. Interactions between digoxin and potassium-sparing diuretics. Clin. Pharmacol. Ther. 33:418–423, 1983.
2. Waldorff, S., Berning, J., Buch, J., and Steiness, E. Systolic time intervals during spironolactone treatment of digitalized and non-digitalized patients with ischaemic heart disease. Eur. J. Clin. Pharmacol. 21:269–273, 1982.
3. Brown, D.D., Spector, R., and Juhl, R.P. Drug interactions with digoxin. Drugs 20:198–206, 1980.
4. Maletzky, B.M. Enhancing the efficacy of lithium treatment by combined use with diuretics and low sodium diets: a preliminary report. J. Clin. Psychiatry 40:317–322, 1979.
5. Himmelhoch, J.M., Poust, R.I., Mallinger, A.G., Hanin, I., and Neil, J.F. Adjustment of lithium dose during lithium chlorothiazide therapy. Clin. Pharmacol. Ther. 22:225–227, 1977.
6. Levenson, D.J., Simmons, C.E., and Brenner, B.M. Arachidonic acid metabolism, prostaglandins and the kidney. Am. J. Med. 72:354–374, 1982.

7. Steiness, E., and Waldorff, S. Different interactions of indomethacin and sulindac with thiazides in hypertension. Br. Med. J. 285:1702–1703, 1982.
8. Patak, R.V., Mookerjee, B.K., Bentzel, C.J., Hysert, P.E., Babej Milos, and Lee, J.B. Antagonism of the effects of furosemide by indomethacin in normal and hypertensive man. Prostaglandins 10:649–659, 1975.
9. Watkins, J., Abbott, E.C., Hensby, C.N., Webster, J., and Dollerty, C.T. Attenuation of hypotensive effect of propranolol and diuretics by indomethacin. Br. Med. J. 281:702–705, 1980.
10. Attallah, A.A. Interaction of prostaglandins with diuretics. Prostaglandins 18:369–375, 1979.
11. Planas, R., Arroyo, V., Rimola, A., Perez-Ayuso, R.M., and Rodes, J. Acetylsalicyclic acid suppresses the renal hemodynamic effect and reduces the diuretic action of furosemide in cirrhosis with ascites. Gastroent. 84:247–252, 1983.
12. Favre, L., Glasson, P., and Vallotton, M.B. Reversible acute renal failure from combined triamterene and indomethacin. Ann. Intern. Med. 96:317–320, 1982.
13. Orr, L. Potentiation of myelosuppression from cancer chemotherapy and thiazide diuretics. Drug Intel. Clin. Pharm. 15:967–969, 1981.
14. Malach, M., and Berman, N. Furosemide and chloral hydrate. Adverse interaction. J. Amer. Med. Assoc. 232:638–639, 1975.
15. Pevonka, M.P., Yost, R.L., Marks, R.G., Howell, W.S., and Stewart, R.B. Interaction of chloral hydrate and furosemide. Drug Intel. Clin. Pharm. 11:332–335, 1977.
16. Petrick, R.J., Kronacher, N., and Aloena, V. Interaction between warfarin and ethacrynic acid. J. Amer. Med. Assoc. 231:843–844, 1975.
17. O'Reilly, R.A. Spironolactone and warfarin interaction. Clin. Pharmacol. Ther. 27:198–201, 1980.
18. Papanicolaou, N., McNeil, B.J., Funkenstein, H.H., and Sudarsky, L.R. Abnormal cisternogram associated with Diamox therapy. J. Nucl. Med. 19:501–503, 1978.
19. Stockley, I. Drug interactions, 1981, Boston, Blackwell Scientific Publications.
20. Lawson, D.H., Tilstone, W.J., Gray, J.M.B., and Srivastava, P.K. Effect of furosemide on the pharmacokinetics of gentamicin in patients. J. Clin. Pharmacol. 22:254–258, 1982.
21. Markman, M., and Trump, D.L. Nephrotoxicity with cisplatin and antihypertensive medications. Ann. Intern. Med. 96:257 (letter), 1982.
22. Bridgman, J.F., Rosen, S.M., and Thorp, J.M. Complications during clofibrate treatment of nephrotic syndrome hyperlipoproteinemia. Lancet 2:506–509, 1972.
23. Ahmad, S. Renal insensitivity to furosemide caused by chronic anticonvulsant therapy. Brit. Med. J. 3:657–659, 1974.
24. Brater, D.C. Effects of probenecid on furosemide response. Clin. Pharmacol. Ther. 24:548–554, 1978.
25. Wood, A.J.J., and Feely, J. Pharmacokinetic drug interactions with propranolol. Clin. Pharmacokin. 8:253–262, 1983.
26. Conlon, P.F., Grambau, G.R., Johnson, C.E., and Weg, J.G. Effect of intravenous furosemide on serum theophylline concentration. Am. J. Hosp. Pharm. 38:1345–1347, 1981.

27. Young, J.L., Boswell, R.B., and Nies, A.S. Severe allopurinol hypersensitivity. Association with thiazides and prior renal compromise. Arch. Intern. Med. 134:553–558, 1974.
28. Lang, P.G. Severe hypersensitivity reactions to allopurinol. So. Med. J. 72:1361–1368, 1979.
29. Kauffman, R.E., and Azarnoff, D.L. Effect of colestipol on gastrointestinal absorption of chlorothiazide in man. Clin. Pharmacol. Ther. 14:886–890, 1973.
30. Bellward, G.D., Warren, P.M., Howald, W., Axelson, J.E., and Abbott, F.S. Methadone maintenance: effect of urinary pH on renal clearance in chronic high and low doses. Clin. Pharmacol. Ther. 22:92–99, 1977.

chapter

14

Determination of Diuretic Sites and Mechanisms of Action

An Outline of Methodology Employed

Jules B. Puschett, M.D.

The determination of those sites within the nephron at which diuretics are active in impairing sodium reabsorption is based largely upon the results of indirect observations obtained in human subjects (1, 2). These findings have been compared and contrasted with more direct measurements performed in the experimental animal utilizing micropuncture methodology (3, 4) and the isolated tubular perfusion technique (5). The majority of the information available, however, is derived from human studies, in which the classical clearance technique has been utilized. This type of investigation represents a "black box" approach to the analysis of kidney function. In employing this methodology, one monitors the amount of a given ion or other solute (per unit time) that the kidney tubular systems of the subject or patient are receiving (the filtered load). In addition, the urinary excretion is measured, and then these two determinations are subtracted from each other to evaluate the transport alterations induced by diuretic agents. The data to be presented in this chapter have been provided largely by the examination of diuretic site of action utilizing the clearance technique. Where appropriate, information obtained from other experimental observations has been included. A comprehensive and encyclopedic compilation has not been attempted. Rather, an outline of important principles and key examples is presented.

The analysis of drug site and mechanism of action involves an evaluation of the drug's effects on principally four functions of the kidney: 1) the urinary diluting and concentrating mechanisms; 2) the pattern of anionic (principally phosphate and bicarbonate) excretion; 3) acid excretion; and 4) renal potassium handling.

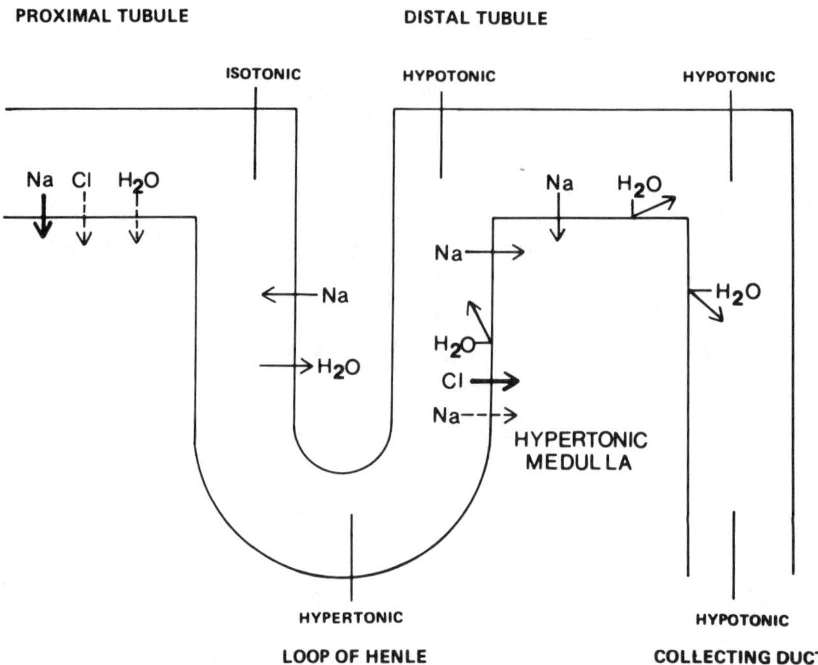

Figure 14-1. Tubular fluid transport throughout the nephron is depicted in the absence of antidiuretic hormone (ADH). *Reproduced from J. Clin. Pharm. 21:564–574, 1981, with permission of the editors.*

Diuretic Effects on Concentration and Dilution

The investigation of diuretic effects on the concentrating and diluting mechanisms of the kidney takes advantage of the fact that the thick or outer medullary portion of the ascending limb of the loop of Henle is the major site at which urinary dilution occurs (Figure 14-1) and that this nephron segment, along with the collecting duct, is responsible for the elaboration of a concentrated urine. Therefore, any diuretic agent which inhibits sodium chloride reabsorption in the ascending limb of the loop of Henle will cause an interference with the ability of the kidney to generate solute-free water. The latter is a function of urinary dilution and represents its quantitative aspect. In the hydrated subject, urine flow rate (V) is equal to the solute clearance (Cosm) plus the solute-free water clearance (CH_2O). Since solute clearance is equal to UosmV/Posm, and since all of the latter parameters can be measured, we can solve for CH_2O as follows: $CH_2O = V - Cosm$. Normal urinary dilution depends upon four factors: 1) normal (or near normal) glomerular filtration rate (GFR); 2) normal function of the proximal tubule so that normal amounts of salt and water reach the diluting sites (located in the ascending limb of the loop of Henle and the early distal convoluted tubule; see Chapter 1); 3) normal loop of Henle function; and 4) suppression of antidiuretic hormone (ADH) release.

Normally, the proximal tubule reabsorbs approximately 60–70% of the filtered load of sodium chloride and fluid. If, for example, diuretic administration has resulted in marked volume contraction, the proximal tubule will respond by increasing its reabsorption of ions and fluid. Therefore, distal delivery of salt and water will be compromised and CH_2O will be reduced. Also, if the reabsorption of sodium chloride at the level of the loop of Henle is interfered with, CH_2O will be reduced in a major way. An example of this effect is shown in Figure 14-2. In this study (6), performed in a hydrated subject undergoing a maximal water diuresis, CH_2O was substantially reduced by ethacrynic acid (Edecrin), implicating the loop of Henle as a major site of action of the drug.

If, on the other hand, a diuretic were to act in the proximal tubule to inhibit sodium chloride and fluid reabsorption, the effect would be to present more ions and water to the diluting sites. The expected result would be that more sodium would be transported from the tubular contents, more tubular water would be "freed" of its solute and, therefore, CH_2O should rise. An example of this sort of action by a diuretic is presented in Figure 14-3 in which acetazolamide (Diamox) was given intravenously to a subject undergoing a sustained water diuresis. Following the drug's administration, urine flow rate (V) rose by roughly the same amount as CH_2O increased, with very little change in solute clearance (Cosm). These data suggest that acetazolamide has interfered with proximal tubular reabsorption (utilizing V here as an indication of distal delivery)* and that end-proximal tubular contents (electrolytes and water) have been delivered downstream to the diluting sites, augmenting free water generation, as measured by the rise in CH_2O. Furthermore, acetazolamide might be expected to have this effect for two reasons: 1) *in vitro*, it is a potent inhibitor of the enzyme carbonic anhydrase (7, 8) and 2) the proximal nephron is the locus of the bulk of bicarbonate "reabsorption."

When the subject (or experimental animal) is hydropenic, not only is there no CH_2O formed, but water is abstracted from the collecting duct, forming a concentrated urine. The circumstances which provide for this physiological sequence of events include mild serum hypertonicity as a stimulus to the hypothalamus for the secretion of ADH, and the nephron effect of the hormone, resulting in the hydroosmotic flow of water from

*During maximal water diuresis, fluid transport in the distal convoluted tubule and collecting duct are minimal because ADH release is suppressed. Consequently, with the exception of water transport from the descending limb (which is not of significance quantitatively) V can be used as an indicator of delivery of fluid out of the proximal tubule.

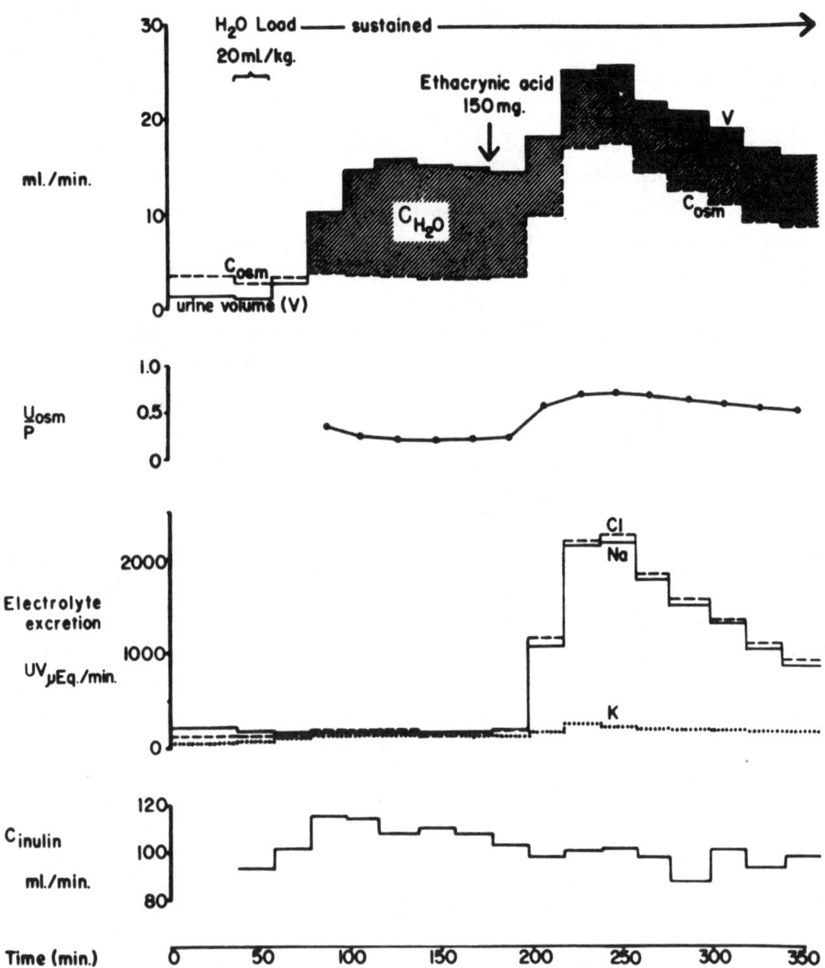

Figure 14-2. The effects of ethacrynic acid administration on free water clearance (CH_2O), urine flow rate (V), and solute clearance (Cosm) in a subject undergoing a maximal water diuresis. *Reproduced from J. Clin. Invest. 43:201–216. 1964, with permission of the editors.*

the tubular lumen into the hypertonic medullary interstitium (Figure 14-4). The gradient which acts as the force for the water reabsorption is provided by the active transport of chloride (with accompanying sodium ions) from the loop of Henle and the reabsorption of urea from the loop of Henle and the collecting duct. Therefore, any diuretic agent which has a major effect on loop of Henle transport processes will interfere with the establishment of the hypertonic medullary interstitium and will obviate the gradient which results in solute free water abstraction (the symbol for

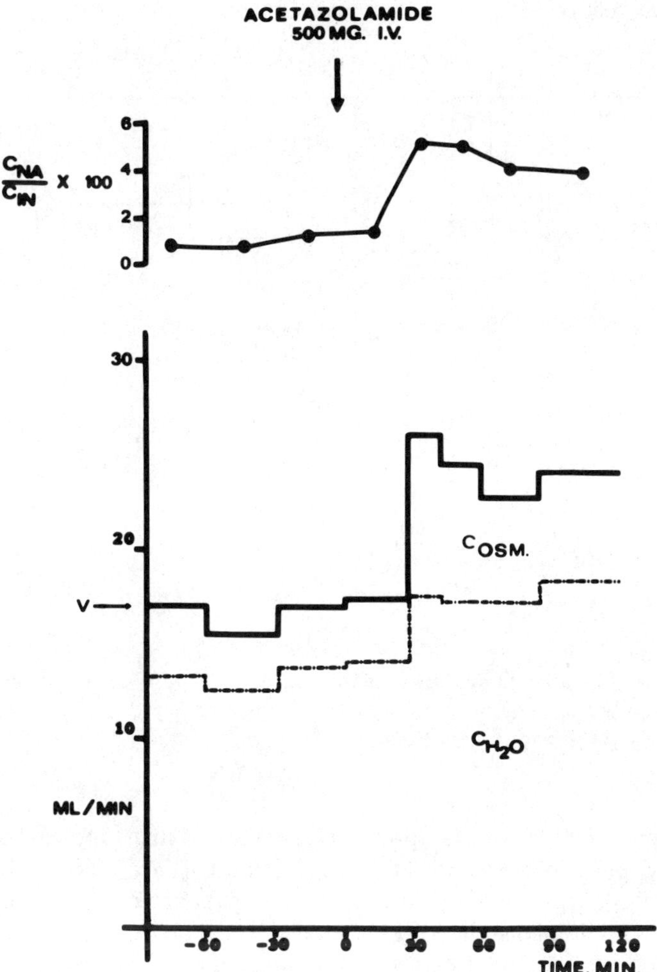

Figure 14-3. The influence of the intravenous administration of acetazolamide (Diamox) on percentage sodium excretion ($C_{Na}/C_{In} \times 100$), osmolal clearance (Cosm), urine flow rate (V) and free water clearance (CH_2O). The drug was given to a normal subject undergoing maximal water diuresis. *Reproduced from J. Clin. Pharm. 21:564–574, 1981, with permission of the editors.*

which is T^cH_2O) from the collecting duct. An example of such a diuretic is ethacrynic acid. When given to hydropenic normal human subjects undergoing saline diuresis, ethacrynic acid dramatically reduced T^cH_2O (Figure 14-5). These data, taken together with the studies of the effects of the drug on CH_2O (see above), strongly implicate the ascending limb of the loop of Henle as a major site of the drug's natriuretic action (6).

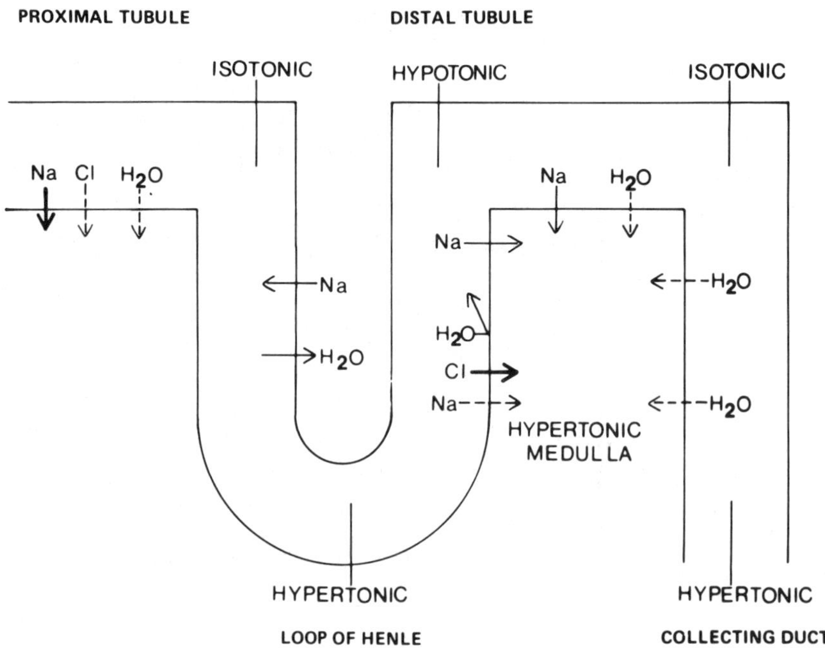

Figure 14-4. Tubular fluid transport throughout the nephron is depicted in the presence of antidiuretic hormone (ADH). *Reproduced from J. Clin. Pharm. 21:564–574, 1981, with permission of the editors.*

In some cases, diuretics appear to have more than one site of action, resulting in combined effects on CH_2O and T^cH_2O. Two noteworthy examples are bumetanide (Bumex) and metolazone (Zaroxolyn, Diulo). In the hydrated human subject, bumetanide caused no change in CH_2O while increasing both V and Cosm (9). When studied during hydropenia, the drug virtually abolished T^cH_2O (10). These observations can be explained if bumetanide inhibits (sodium) chloride transport in the loop of Henle but also impairs sodium reabsorption in the proximal tubule. Thus, during water diuresis, the proximal effect of the drug, leading to increased distal delivery of salt and water, offsets the inhibitory action of the drug on CH_2O. The effect of the diuretic on T^cH_2O verifies its action in the ascending limb of the loop of Henle, and the performance of micropuncture studies in the dog has verified a proximal tubular effect of bumetanide (11).

During sustained maximal water diuresis, the ascending limb of the loop of Henle represents the site at which most of the free water is generated. However, as can be seen in Figure 14-1 (see also site 3, Figure 1-2, Chapter 1), there is an additional locus of free water formation in the early portion

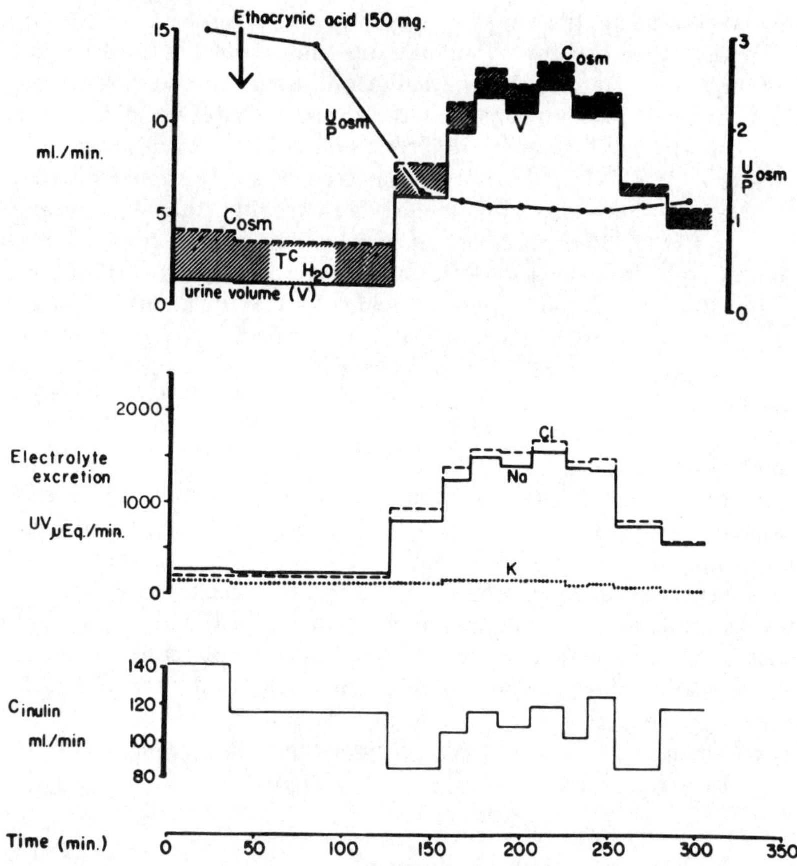

Figure 14-5. The effects of ethacrynic acid, given to a normal subject undergoing maximal water diuresis, on the abstraction of solute-free water from the collecting duct (T^cH_2O), osmolal clearance (Cosm) and urine flow rate (V). C_{inulin} represents the estimation of glomerular filtration rate by the measurement of the clearance of inulin. *Reproduced with permission of the editors from J. Clin. Invest. 43:201–216, 1964.*

of the distal convoluted tubule. The latter site has a limited ability (especially compared to the ascending limb of the loop of Henle) to form solute-free water. Therefore, a drug which impairs sodium transport in this nephron segment would interfere in a less major way with urinary dilution, and consequently would decrease CH_2O less than an agent which had a profound effect on loop of Henle NaCl reabsorption. Such a drug should, therefore, have no effect on T^cH_2O which, as described above, is a loop of Henle function. As a group, the thiazides seem to act largely at the transport site in the early distal convolution, since, although the data are somewhat conflicting, they appear to reduce CH_2O modestly, but do not affect T^cH_2O. These findings essentially rule out an effect in the ascending limb of the loop of Henle (12, 13). Metolazone, administered during water diuresis, caused a mild but consistent reduction in CH_2O, yet did not alter T^cH_2O in hydropenic human subjects undergoing a hypertonic saline diuresis (13). Metolazone was also suspected of an additional proximal effect because it caused a phosphaturia and resulted in only a modest decline in CH_2O. Phosphate is an ion which is largely reabsorbed proximally (see also discussion of anionic transport, below). Accordingly, micropuncture studies were performed in the dog to determine if this thesis regarding a proximal action could be verified. Indeed, when there was little or no fall in GFR (and, therefore, in filtered sodium load), metolazone could be demonstrated to inhibit proximal sodium, fluid and phosphate reabsorption (14).

Examination of transport with the isolated tubule technique (15) has provided two important advantages over the clearance and micropuncture methodologies. First, it obviates the effects of alterations in renal hemodynamics (renal blood flow and GFR) and in hormonal status which may be caused by diuretics when studied *in vivo*. Second, this technique allows an evaluation of the transport properties of defined nephron segments, some of which are inaccessible to micropuncture. Thus, for example, examination of the isolated thick ascending limb with this methodology first uncovered the information that chloride is the actively transported ion, and verified that chloride transport is inhibited by the loop blockers in a major way (15).

Diuretic Effects on Anionic Excretion

The majority of phosphate reabsorption and a large proportion of bicarbonate reabsorption (estimated at 80–90%) have been determined to occur in the proximal nephron (16). Therefore, the pattern of excretion of these anions has been utilized as a "marker" of proximal tubular effects by diuretic agents. Although the impairment of proximal tubular transport frequently results in both a phosphaturia and a bicarbonate diuresis, the latter are not inevitable consequences of the former (13, 14). This is because proximally rejected phosphate and bicarbonate ions do have opportunities to be reabsorbed at more distal sites in the nephron. However, not only can the proximal and whole kidney effects of diuretic drugs on these anions be dissociated, but it is also possible to inhibit the transport of one ion without an effect on the other. An example of this is provided by recent studies of bumetanide (Bumex) in the dog, utilizing the micropuncture technique combined with clearance measurements (17). In this investigation, the diuretic inhibited proximal bicarbonate but not phosphate reabsorption.

The key to understanding diuretic drug effects on proximal anionic reabsorption probably has to do with an appreciation of the mechanism(s) by which these agents act. The most phosphaturic of the diuretics is acetazolamide, a drug which owes its natriuretic capabilities to its capacity for carbonic anhydrase inhibition (8). Since the enzyme carbonic anhydrase is involved in a major way in the reclamation of bicarbonate by the proximal nephron, any agent which interferes with this process will cause a bicarbonate diuresis (7). Furthermore, alterations in tubular pH seem to be important in determining the magnitude of phosphate transport. Acetazolamide and other carbonic anhydrase inhibitors alkalinize the tubular contents. In an alkaline medium, phosphate excretion, rather than reabsorption, appears to be favored (16). The basis, then, for the tendency of acetazolamide (7) and chlorothiazide (13) to cause both a phosphaturia and a bicarbonate diuresis appears to be in the similarities of their chemical structures (Figure 14-6). Both of these drugs possess an unsubstituted sulfonamido ($-SO_2NH_2$) group, the chemical characteristic necessary for carbonic anhydrase inhibitory action.

However, the fact that a drug has this chemical grouping does not automatically confer carbonic anhydrase activity. Thus, for example, metolazone's proximal effect does not seem to be related to an ability to inhibit the enzyme (17), nor does either bumetanide (11) or peritanide (18) act proximally by this mechanism (17).

Diuretic Effects on Acid Excretion

In addition to the reabsorption of bicarbonate, the body rids itself of the daily burden of hydrogen ions resulting from the metabolism of food stuffs by excreting them. Hydrogen may be excreted either attached to urinary buffers (the major one of which is phosphate) or by the addition of hydrogen ion to ammonia (NH_3) gas which freely diffuses across the renal tubular cell membrane from the blood, into the tubular lumen. The former of these two processes is called titratable acid excretion and the latter, ammonium excretion. Hydrogen ion excretion is given by the formula:

$U_{H^+}V = U_{TA}V + U_{NH_4^+}V - U_{HCO_3^-}V$ (19), in which $U_{H^+}V$ is net acid excretion, $U_{TA}V$ represents titratable acid excretion, and $U_{NH_4^+}V$ and $U_{HCO_3^-}V$ are the absolute excretion rates of ammonium and bicarbonate, respectively, each expressed as μEq/min (or, mEq/24 hr).

Observations regarding the effects of diuretics on these parameters are of importance for two reasons: First, they indicate something about the drug's mechanism and site of action within the nephron. Second, information of this kind has implications clinically. That is, it may suggest or explain acid-base disturbances that will or do result from the use of certain diuretics.

Instances of the importance of these observations for both renal

① SULFONAMIDE DERIVATIVES

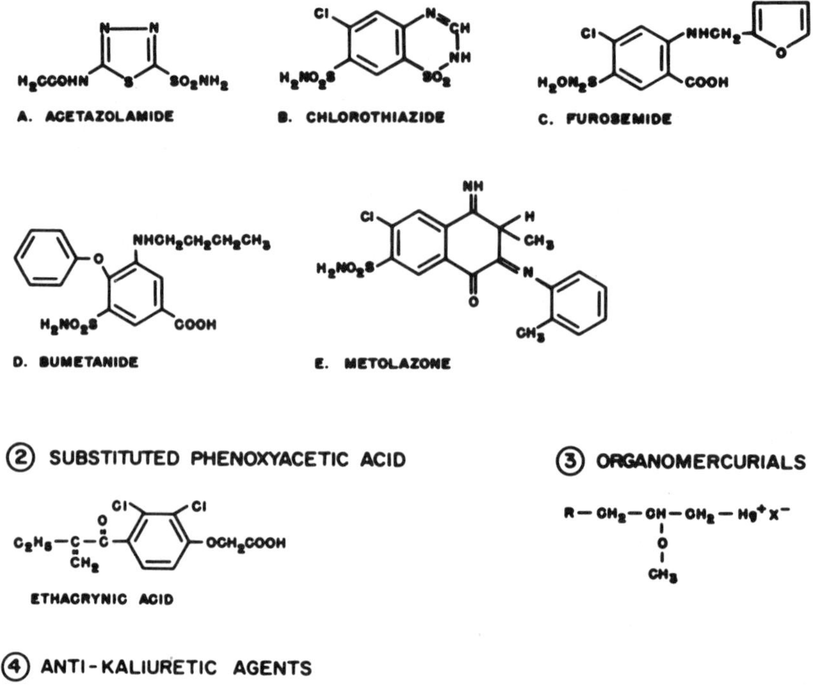

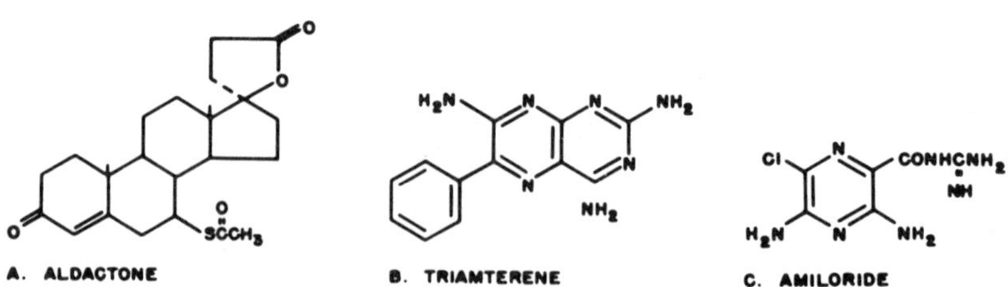

Figure 14-6. Depiction of the chemical structures of the commonly utilized diuretic agents. *Reproduced from J. Clin. Pharm. 21:564–574, 1981, with permission of the editors.*

physiology and clinical medicine abound. For example, the administration of the carbonic anhydrase inhibitor, acetazolamide (Diamox), results in an inhibition of bicarbonate reabsorption, so that bicarbonate excretion (U_{HCO_3}–V, see formula above) increases. With this base loss, net acid excretion (U_{H^+}V) becomes a negative figure. Stated in another way, hydrogen ion accumulates in the body since it is not excreted. This means that with chronic administration of the drug, metabolic acidosis is a real possibility.

Most of the potent diuretics (e.g., furosemide, ethacrynic acid) cause the excretion of relatively more chloride than bicarbonate as the anion which accompanies the excreted sodium cations. Since the increased presentation of sodium to the distal nephron results in an increased exchange of sodium for hydrogen (as well as potassium) ions, hydrogen ion excretion will increase. As noted in the above formula, if either titratable acid or ammonium excretion, or both, increase to a greater extent than does $U_{HCO_3^-}V$, then net acid excretion will increase. If this occurs on a daily basis, then the patient will go into negative hydrogen ion balance and there is the likelihood that metabolic alkalosis will result. Indeed, the commonest acid-base disturbance noted in diuresed patients is metabolic alkalosis, usually of the hypokalemic variety.

Finally, some agents seem to affect both hydrogen and bicarbonate excretion to about the same extent. Accordingly, urine pH would be expected not to change after administration of the drug, and net acid excretion by the body should not change. An example of just such a situation is that represented by the acute infusion of bumetanide (10). Shown in Figure 14-7 are data obtained in a representative study in which the drug was given intravenously to a normal volunteer and the parameters of acid excretion described above were measured. The increase in urinary flow rate and increased activity of the sodium-hydrogen exchange sites in the distal nephron, as well as a modest inhibition of bicarbonate excretion not mediated by carbonic anhydrase inhibition (9, 11), resulted in mild increments in $U_{TA}V$ and $U_{NH^+}V$ which were offset by a modest rise in $U_{HCO_3^-}V$. The net result was that $U_{H^+}V$ and urinary pH did not change (10).

Effects of Diuretics on Potassium Handling by the Nephron

According to current concepts, potassium is virtually completely reabsorbed by the end of the loop of Henle and that which appears in the final urine is that secreted by the distal tubule and early collecting duct (20). Some recycling of potassium betwen the descending limb of the loop of Henle and collecting duct appears to occur, but probably does not account for any major addition of potassium to the final urine. Accordingly, potassium excretion can be increased by inhibiting its reabsorption and/or by enhancing its secretion, both of which processes may play a role in diuretic-induced kaliuresis (see also the discussion of this matter in Chapter 1). Furthermore, as a general rule, diuretics which inhibit sodium transport at any site upstream of the sodium-hydrogen-potassium exchange sites in the late distal nephron will present more sodium for reabsorption at those sites. Consequently, the more potent a diuretic is in

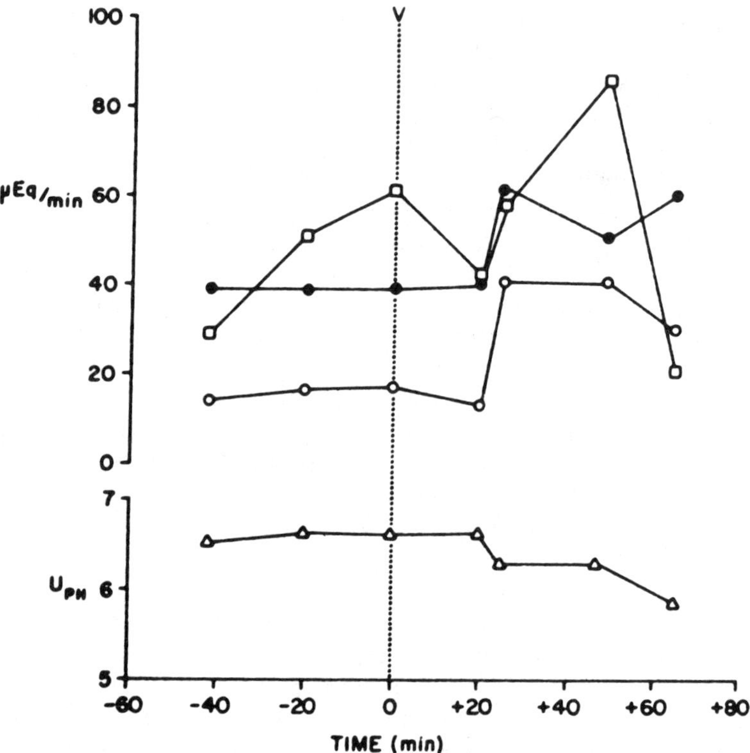

Figure 14-7. Effects of bumetanide (administered at time zero) on acid excretion in a normal subject. $U_{H+}V$ = net acid excretion; $U_{TA}V$ = titratable and excretion; $U_{NH_4^+}V$ and $U_{HCO_3^-}V$ = absolute excretion rates of ammonium and bicarbonate, respectively. Key: ○——○ = $U_{TA}V$, ●——● = $U_{NH_4^+}V$, and □——□ = $U_{HCO_3^-}V$. *Reproduced from J. Pharm. Exp. Ther. 201:251–258, 1977, with permission of the editors.*

inhibiting sodium reabsorption, the greater the kaliuretic tendency of that drug (cf. Chapter 1 and Figure 1-3).

A drug which acts on the nephron to reduce potassium excretion will have done so, most likely, by interfering with the secretion of potassium into the tubular fluid at the specialized exchange sites in the late distal nephron. These so-called potassium-sparing agents (Figure 14-6) act via one of two mechanisms: 1) spironolactone (Aldactone) is a competitive inhibitor of aldosterone, and therefore interferes with the usual mineralocorticoid regulation of transport activity at these specialized exchange sites. 2) triamterene (Dyrenium) and amiloride (Midamor) block the secretion of potassium directly. They act on the portion of the sodium-hydrogen-potassium exchange mechanism that functions even in the absence of aldosterone. The transport of potassium effected by these drugs is therefore mineralocorticoid-independent.

In general, therefore, the potassium excretion effects of diuretics are examined largely for two reasons. First, it is generally recognized that the more potent a drug is as a natriuretic agent, the greater will be the tendency for kaliuresis and consequent hypokalemia. Second, certain drugs may have the capacity to interfere with the secretion of potassium into the urine, rendering them potentially helpful as adjunctive agents to minimize potassium loss.

References

1. Seldin, D.R., Eknoyan, G., Suki, W.N., and Rector, F.C., Jr. Localization of diuretic action from the pattern of water and electrolyte excretion, in The Physiology of Diuretic Agents, Ann. N.Y. Acad. Sci. 139:328–343, 1966.
2. Puschett, J.B. Sites and mechanisms of action of diuretics in the kidney. J. Clin. Pharmacol. 21:564–574, 1981.
3. Deetjen, P. Micropuncture studies on site and mode of diuretic action of furosemide. Ann. N.Y. Acad. Sci. 139:408–415, 1966.
4. Ulrich, K.J., Baumann, K., Loeschke, K., Rumrick, G., and Stolte, H. Micropuncture experiments with saluretic sulfonamides. Ann. N.Y. Acad. Sci. 139:416–423, 1966.
5. Burg, M., Stoner, L., Cardinal, J., and Green, N. Furosemide effect on isolated perfused tubules. Am. J. Physiol. 225:119–124, 1973.
6. Goldberg, M., McCurdy, D.K., Foltz, E.L., and Bluemle, L.W., Jr. Effects of ethacrynic acid (a new saluretic agent) on renal diluting and concentrating mechanisms: evidence for site of action in the loop of Henle. J. Clin. Invest. 43:201–216, 1964.
7. Puschett, J.B., and Goldberg, M. The acute effects of furosemide on acid and electrolyte excretion in man. J. Lab. Clin. Med. 71:666–677, 1968.
8. Maren, T.H. Carbonic anhydrase: chemistry, physiology and inhibition. Physiol. Rev. 47:597–781, 1967.
9. Puschett, J.B. Renal effects of bumetanide. J. Clin. Pharmacol. 21:575–580, 1981.
10. Jayakumar, S., and Puschett, J.B. Study of the sites and mechanisms of action of bumetanide in man. J. Pharmacol. Exp. Therap. 201:251–258, 1977.
11. Puschett, J.B., Sylk, D.B., and Teredesai, P.R. Uncoupling of proximal sodium bicarbonate from sodium phosphate transport by bumetanide. Am. J. Physiol. 235:F60–F68, 1980.
12. Earley, L.E., Kahn, M., and Orloff, J. The effects of infusion of chlorothiazide on urinary dilution and concentration in the dog. J. Clin. Invest. 40:857–866, 1961.
13. Steinmuller, S.R., and Puschett, J.B. Effects of metholazone in man: comparison with chlorothiazide. Kidney Internat. 1:169–181, 1972.
14. Fernandez, P.C., and Puschett, J.B. Proximal tubular actions of metolazone and chlorothiazide. Am. J. Physiol. 235:904–961, 1973.
15. Burg, M., Grantham, J., Abramow, M., and Orloff, J. Preparation and study of fragments of single rabbit nephrons. Am. J. Physiol. 210:1293–1298, 1966.

16. Puschett, J.B., and Goldberg, M. The relationship between the renal handling of phosphate and bicarbonate in man. J. Lab. Clin. Med. 73:956–969, 1969.
17. Puschett, J.B., Steinmuller, S.R., Rastegar, A., and Fernandez, P. Metolazone: mechanism and sites of action. In, Modern Diuretic Therapy in the Treatment of Cardiovascular and Renal Disease, edited by A.F. Lant and G.M. Wilson, Amsterdam, Excerpta Medica, pp. 168–178, 1973.
18. Winaver, J., Sylk, D.B., Teredesai, P.R., Robertson, J.S., and Puschett, J.B. Dissociative effects of piretanide on proximal tubular PO_4 and HCO_3 transport. Am. J. Physiol. 238:F60–F68, 1980.
19. Elkinton, J.R., McCurdy, D.K., and Buckalew, V.M., Jr. Hydrogen ion and the kidney. In: Renal Disease, 2nd edition, 1967 (editor: D.A.K. Black), Philadelphia, F.A. Davis Co., pp. 110–135.
20. Wright, F.S., and Giebisch, G. Renal potassium transport: contributions of individual nephron segments and populations. Am. J. Physiol. 235:F515–F527, 1978.

PART

II

APPENDICES

Thomas O. Pitts, M.D.

The tables of the Appendices to *The Diuretic Manual* are designed to provide the reader with a reference summarizing many of the important and useful details regarding therapy with the currently available diuretic agents. Appendix 1 compares the relative potency of the various classes of diuretics and provides information on dosages and pharmacologic parameters of certain specific drugs in each class. Appendix 2 lists the site(s) of action of each class of diuretic and, where known, the mechanism. In choosing combination diuretic therapy, the physician should be aware of the site(s) and mechanism(s) of action of the agents selected, so that a rational choice of drugs can be made. Appendix 3 summarizes briefly the indications for therapy with diuretics and directs the reader to the appropriate chapters in the book which provide a discussion of the particular disorder under consideration. Appendix 4 is a list of the generic and corresponding brand names of the commonly used drugs in each class. In addition, the frequently prescribed combination diuretics and diuretic/antihypertensive agents are indexed alphabetically by brand names in Appendix 5. The reader is reminded that combination drugs are not indicated as initial therapy for hypertension since the dose of each drug must be optimized individually for each patient.

The thiazide and thiazide-like group includes the prototype agents chlorothiazide and hydrochlorothiazide as well as several structurally similar sulfonamide derivatives such as chlorthalidone and quinethazone (see Appendix 4 and Table 5-6). Typically, agents in this classification: 1) exert their effects on sodium reabsorption in the early distal tubule (see Appendix 2), 2) provide a maximal fractional excretion of sodium of 5–8% of the filtered load, 3) are mildly to moderately kaliuretic and 4) are ineffective when the glomerular filtration rate falls below about 25% of normal. Metolazone is an agent similar in potency to the thiazides but remains an effective diuretic even in states of moderate renal insufficiency. The combination of metolazone with a loop blocker provides a particularly potent diuretic regimen for cases of resistant edema. The duration of action of metolazone approaches 24–36 hr when maximal dosage is given.*

Carbonic anhydrase inhibitors produce a bicarbonate diuresis and achieve a maximal fractional excretion of sodium slightly less than that seen with the thiazides. They are most commonly used for the treatment of glaucoma and may be given intravenously when this disturbance is severe.

*Except as mentioned, the thiazide diuretics are interchangeable; no one congener offers any particular advantage over another. The author suggests that the practicing physician familiarize himself with the use of one or two of these agents and use them exclusively. For this reason, most chapters describe the use of hydrochlorothiazide; chlorothiazide or any of the other agents of this group listed in Appendix 4 could be substituted. Note that it would be irrational to switch practices, for example, to bendroflumethiazide in the hope of alleviating a complication or side effect of hydrochlorothiazide therapy.

The dosages required for ophthalmologic treatment generally exceed those used for diuresis. With chronic use, these agents may produce metabolic acidosis, a condition which inhibits the renal effect of such drugs. Since other, more potent, diuretics are available today, carbonic anhydrase inhibitors are not often used for the control of edematous states.

The "loop blockers," furosemide, ethacrynic acid and bumetanide, are the most potent of available diuretics, producing a maximal sodium excretion of 20–25% of the filtered load. They are available in oral and intravenous forms, and when necessary can be given more than once daily. They produce marked increments in potassium excretion, and thus, may produce hypokalemia. They are effective in states of moderate to severe renal insufficiency and may induce or worsen azotemia. These drugs are potentially ototoxic and may produce hearing impairment when given in frequent and/or high doses, especially if administered by rapid intravenous infusion. Thus, therapy with loop blockers should be individualized, and cautious follow-up of electrolyte and renal functional status is imperative.

The antikaliuretic or "potassium sparing" agents include spironolactone, triamterene, and amiloride. These drugs produce a maximal fractional sodium excretion of only 2–3% of filtered load and are not generally used alone as principal agents for antihypertensive or edema therapy. Hyperkalemia is a potential complication of therapy, and is especially likely in states of azotemia. In most patients, these drugs are used in combination with the thiazide/thiazide-like or loop blocking agents to attempt to prevent hypokalemia. Spironolactone is a particularly unique agent in that it directly inhibits the renal tubular action of aldosterone (see Appendix 3) and, thus, is useful in states of aldosterone excess (e.g., in cirrhosis and certain hypertensive disorders). The effect of spironolactone is gradual in onset so that dosage changes should not be instituted more frequently than once each 2–3 days at the earliest.

Mercurial diuretics were once effective and popular agents for the therapy of edematous disorders. However, the safer and more effective loop blockers have made these drugs obsolete.

Mannitol is a sugar which is relatively inert, is freely filtered by the glomerulus and is not appreciably reabsorbed by the renal tubule. It, therefore, produces a diuresis by osmotically inhibiting tubular fluid and sodium reabsorption. The resultant urinary flow and sodium excretion vary directly with the administered load. In addition, urine osmolality approaches isotonicity as solute excretion and urine flow increase. While mannitol acts all along the tubule to inhibit fluid reabsorption its inhibition of sodium excretion occurs primarily in the ascending limb of the loop of Henle. This drug, which must be given intravenously, is used as a continuous infusion to maintain urinary flow in certain special circumstances (for example, in post-operative or peri-operative periods, see Chapter 7). Also, it is occasionally given in single doses for acute glaucoma, cerebral edema, in preparation for ophthalmologic or neurosurgical procedures and for prophylaxis of acute renal failure (see Chapter 7). It may precipitate volume overload in susceptible patients and may produce hyponatremia and hyperosmolarity. Its use should be avoided in patients with advanced renal insufficiency.

APPENDIX 1. Relative Potency of Diuretic Drugs; Onset and Duration of Action

Class	Total Daily Dose Range	Dose Frequency per Day	Onset after Oral Dose (hr)	Onset after IV Dose	Duration of effect (oral)
THIAZIDES/THIAZIDE-LIKE:					
Chlorothiazide	0.5–2 gm	1–2	2	15 min	6–12 hr
Hydrochlorothiazide	50–100 mg	1–2	2	—	6–12 hr
Chlorthalidone	25–50 mg	1	2	—	48–72 hr
METOLAZONE					
	2.5–20 mg	1	1	—	12–24 hr
CARBONIC ANHYDRASE INHIBITORS:					
Acetazolamide	(as a diuretic agent) 250–1000 mg	1–2	1–2	30–60 min	8–12 hr
	(for glaucoma) 250–1500 mg	3–6			
LOOP-BLOCKERS:[a]					
Furosemide	20–240 mg	1–2	0.5	5 min	6–8 hr (2–3 hr IV)
Ethacrynic acid	50–250 mg	1–2	0.5	5 min	6–8 hr (3 hr IV)
Bumetanide	0.5–2.0 mg	1–2	0.5	5 min	4–6 hr (2–3 hr IV)
ANTIKALIURETIC AGENTS:					
Spironolactone	25–400 mg	1–4	48–72	—	3–4 days after cessation of therapy
Triamterene	100–300 mg	1–2	2–4	—	7–9 hr
Amiloride	5–10 mg	1	2	—	24 hr
MERCURIALS					
	0.5–2.0 ml	3 ×/wk	—IM only—		12–24 hr
OSMOTIC AGENTS					
Mannitol	50–200 mg	variable	—IV only—		

[a]Equipotent doses of these three drugs are: furosemide 40 mg, bumetanide 1 mg and ethacrynic acid 50 mg.

APPENDIX 1 *(continued)*

Maximal fractional sodium excretion (percent of filtered load)	Comments
5–8	Long-acting thiazides (e.g., quinethazone & chlorthalidone) produce hypokalemia more predictably than shorter-acting agents.
5–8	Thiazides are ineffective in the presence of renal insufficiency.
5–8	
5–8	This drug is similar in potency to thiazides, but unlike thiazides, it is effective in states of renal insufficiency. Use with loop blockers provides an extremely potent diuretic action in patients with resistant edema.
3–5	Ophthalmologic dosage exceeds that required for maximal diuretic effect. Renal effect may become blunted by presence of metabolic acidosis due to the drug or by other clinical situations in which metabolic acidosis is present. Effective for glaucoma even in patients with renal insufficiency.
20–25	Dosage of agents in this group is best determined by titration of patients on an individual basis. These drugs are markedly kaliuretic and are effective in states of renal insufficiency. Frequent and/or high
20–25	bolus (IV) doses may result in ototoxicity.[b]
20–25	
2–3	Effect of spironolactone is dependent on presence of aldosterone, and is gradual in onset and reversal. Thus, dosage changes should be done only at 1–2 wk intervals.
2–3	These agents act independently of the patient's aldosterone status. They
2–3	may produce azotemia, hyperkalemia and/or metabolic acidosis.
15–20	These once-useful drugs have become obsolete with the development of the newer loop-diuretics.
variable	As solute load increases, urine flow and sodium excretion rise proportionally and urine osmolality approaches isotonicity. A constant infusion of 50–200 gm over 24 hr in the volume replete patient usually maintains urine flow at 30–50 cc/hr. For acute glaucoma, cerebral edema, and preparation for ocular or neurosurgery, the usual dosage is 1.5–2 gm/kg over .5–1 hr. Generally a 50–100 gm slow IV bolus is used for prophylaxis of acute renal failure at the time of the potentially harmful event (surgery, prolonged hypotension, IVP, etc.).

[b]The duration of action of the IV form is prolonged in renal insufficiency.

APPENDIX 2. Classification of Diuretic Agents by Nephron Site and Mechanism of Action*

Agent	Major Nephron Site of Action	Additional (minor) Site of Action	Presumed Mechanism at Major Site of Action
THIAZIDE /THIAZIDE-LIKE	Early distal tubule (may include cortical portion of the ascending limb of the loop of Henle)	Proximal tubule[a,b]	Primary sodium reabsorption inhibition, mechanism unknown
METOLAZONE	Early distal tubule	Proximal tubule[a,c]	Unknown
CARBONIC ANHYDRASE INHIBITORS			
Acetazolamide	Proximal tubule	Distal tubule[d]	Inhibition of carbonic anhydrase thereby blocking $NaHCO_3^-$ reabsorption
LOOP-BLOCKERS			
Furosemide	Ascending limb of the loop of Henle	Proximal tubule[b]	Unknown
Ethacrynic acid	Ascending limb of the loop of Henle	Proximal tubule	Unknown
Bumetanide	Ascending limb of the loop of Henle	Proximal tubule[e]	Unknown
ANTIKALIURETIC AGENTS			
Spironolactone	Late distal tubule and collecting duct	—	Competitive inhibition of the renal tubular action of aldosterone
Triamterene	Late distal tubule and collecting duct	—	Unknown, direct inhibition of potassium secretion by renal tubular cells
Amiloride	Late distal tubule and collecting duct	—	Unknown
MERCURIALS	Ascending limb of the loop of Henle	Proximal tubule[a]	Rupture of carbon-Hg bond to form mercuric ions which react with thiol and other organic groups at receptor sites in the kidney

[a]Action at this site does not generally contribute to diuresis.
[b]This effect is due to a weak inhibition of carbonic anhydrase, associated with the drug's sulfonamide-like structure.
[c]This action represents inhibition of Na-phosphate coupled transport.
[d]Carbonic anhydrase inhibition occurs throughout the nephron but diuresis occurs primarily due to proximal inhibition.
[e]This effect is unrelated to carbonic anhydrase inhibition, despite the drug's sulfonamide structure.
*The reader is referred to Chapter 1 (and Figure 1-2) for a more complete discussion of sodium reabsorptive sites in the nephron.

APPENDIX 3. Diuretic Indications

Disease State		Discussion
Hypertension:	Primary	Chapter 5
	Secondary	
Edematous states:	Nephrotic syndrome	Chapters 1 and
	Liver disease	3
	Heart failure	4
	Renal failure	7, 8
	Idiopathic edema	1
	Edema 2° to drug therapy: e.g., steroids, estrogens	1
Renal stone formers		Chapter 6
Acute renal failure		Chapter 7
Metabolic disturbances:	Syndrome of inappropriate ADH secretion and other hyponatremic states	Chapter 9
	Diabetes insipidus	Chapter 9
	Hypercalcemia	Chapter 6
Miscellaneous conditions:	Prophylaxis for acute renal failure; pretreatment for angiographic dye studies; surgical/trauma cases; pigmenturic states.	Chapter 7
	Cerebral edema	Appendix 1
	Glaucoma[a]	Appendix 1
	Adjunctive therapy in epilepsy[a]	

[a]Carbonic anhydrase inhibitors used for effects other than diuresis.

APPENDIX 4. Generic and Brand Names of Some Commonly Prescribed Diuretic Agents[a]

Class	Generic Name	Brand Names
Thiazides/thiazides-like	Chlorothiazide	Diuril
	Hydrochlorothiazide	Esedrix, HydroDiuril, Oretic, Thiuretic
	Benzthiazide	Exna, Aquatag, Aquex, Hydrex
	Bendroflumethiazide	Naturetin
	Hydroflumethiazide	Saluron, Diucardin
	Methyclothiazide	Aquatensen, Enduron
	Cyclothiazide	Anhydron, Fluidil
	Trichlormethiazide	Naqua, Metahydrin
	Polythiazide	Renese
	Chlorthalidone	Hygroton
	Quinethazone	Hydromox
Metolazone	Metolazone	Zaroxolyn, Diulo
Carbonic anhydrase inhibitors	Acetazolamide	Diamox
Loop blockers	Furosemide	Lasix
	Ethacrynic acid	Edecrin
	Bumetanide	Bumex
Antikaliuretics	Spironolactone	Aldactone
	Triamterene	Dyrenium
	Amiloride	Midamor

[a]Many of these drugs are available in the generic form.

APPENDIX 5. Composition and Dosage of Some Commonly Utilized Diuretic and Antihypertensive Combination Drugs[a]

Brand Name	Generic Names and Drug Dosages	
DIURETIC DRUG COMBINATIONS		
Aldactazide	Spironolactone 25 mg	Hydrochlorothiazide 25 mg
Dyazide	Triamterene 50 mg	Hydrochlorothiazide 25 mg
Moduretic	Amiloride 5 mg	Hydrochlorothiazide 50 mg
DIURETIC/ANTIHYPERTENSIVE DRUGS		
Aldoclor 150/250	Chlorothiazide 150/250 mg	Methyldopa 150/250 mg
Aldoril 15/25/D30/D50	Hydrochlorothiazide 15/25/30/50 mg	Methyldopa 250/250/500/500 mg
Apresazide $\frac{25}{25}, \frac{50}{50}, \frac{100}{50}$	Hydrochlorothiazide 25/50/50 mg	Hydralazine 25/50/100 mg
Apresoline-Esedrix	Hydrochlorothiazide 15 mg	Hydralazine 25 mg
Combipres 0.1/0.2	Chlorthalidone 15/15 mg	Clonidine 0.1/0.2 mg
Demi-Regroton	Chlorthalidone 25 mg	Reserpine 0.125 mg
Diupres 250/500	Chlorothiazide 250/500	Reserpine 0.125/0.125 mg
Diutensin	Methyclothiazide 2.5 mg	Cryptenamine 2 mg
Diutensin R	Methyclothiazide 2.5 mg	Reserpine 0.1 mg
Enduronyl/Endur. Forte	Methyclothiazide 5/5 mg	Deserpidine 0.25/0.5 mg
Esimil	Hydrochlorothiazide 25 mg	Quanethidine 10 mg
Hydromox R	Quinethazone 50 mg	Reserpine 0.125 mg
Hydropres 25/50	Hydrochlorothiazide 25/50 mg	Reserpine 0.125/0.125 mg
Inderide $\frac{40}{25}, \frac{80}{25}$	Hydrochlorothiazide 25/25 mg	Propranolol 40/80 mg
Metatensin #2/#4	Trichlormethiazide 2.0/4.0 mg	Reserpine 0.1/0.1 mg
Minizide 1/2/5	Polythiazide 0.5/0.5/0.5 mg	Prazosin 1/2/5 mg
Naquival	Trichlormethiazide 4 mg	Reserpine 0.1 mg
Oreticyl 25/50/ Forte	Hydrochlorothiazide 25/50/25 mg	Deserpidine .125/.125/.25 mg
Rauzide	Bendroflumethiazide 4 mg	Rauwolfia serpentina 50 mg
Regroton	Chlorthalidone 50 mg	Reserpine 0.25 mg
Renese-R	Polythiazide 2.0 mg	Reserpine 0.25 mg
Ropres	Trichlormethiazide 4 mg	Reserpine 0.1 mg
Salutensin	Hydroflumethiazide 50 mg	Reserpine 0.125 mg
Ser-Ap-Es	Hydrochlorothiazide 25 mg	Reserpine 0.1 mg Hydralazine 25 mg
Serpasil-Esedrix #1/#2	Hydrochlorothiazide 25/50 mg	Reserpine 0.1/0.1 mg
Timolide	Hydrochlorothiazide 25 mg	Timolol 10 mg
Unipres	Hydrochlorothiazide 15 mg	Reserpine 0.1 mg Hydralazine 25 mg

[a]Combination agents are not recommended for initial therapy of hypertensive disorders. The dosage of each drug should first be adjusted in the individual patient. Some combinations are available in the generic form.

Index

D

E

I

K

L

M